DIABETES TYPE 2 MADE SIMPLE

A Beginner's Guide to Diabetes

N. Kehseni Markbron

Dear Reader,

Welcome to "Diabetes Type 2 Made Simple," a comprehensive guide designed to demystify the complexities often associated with Diabetes. In these pages, you will find essential insights and a thorough exploration of every aspect of type 2 diabetes. Whether you are newly diagnosed, have been living with diabetes for some time, or are supporting a loved one, this book aims to provide clarity and practicality, providing you with the necessary tools and knowledge to take charge of your health.

This book is more than just a resource—it's a companion on your journey towards wellness. We cover everything from diabetes history and origin to different complications of diabetes explained using illustrative diagrams all presented in an easy-to-understand format. Our goal is to equip you with a solid understanding of diabetes and the confidence to navigate your path to better health.

Join us as we explore the fundamentals of diabetes, debunk common myths, and provide you with up-to-date, evidence-based information. It's time to turn challenges into opportunities and make living with Type 2 diabetes as simple and straightforward as possible. Together, we can pave the way for a healthier, more fulfilling life.

N. Kehseni Markbron

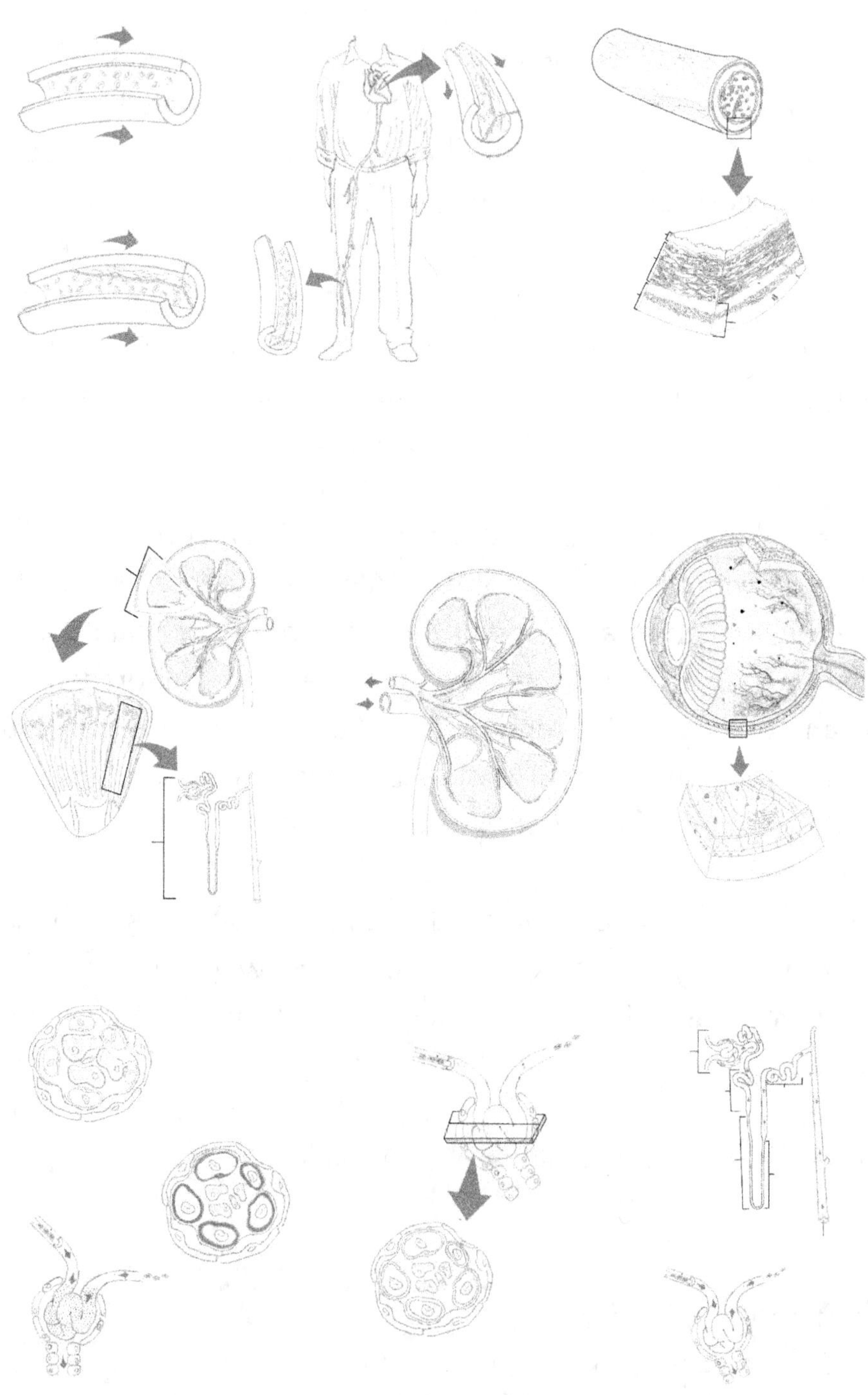

TABLE OF CONTENTS

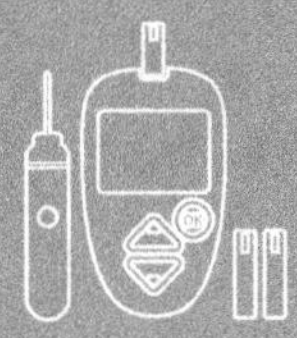

TABLE OF CONTENTS

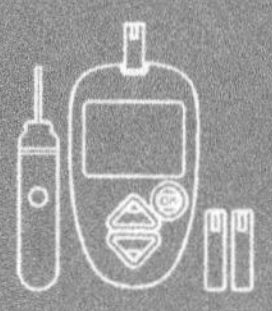

INTRODUCTION

ORIGIN

&

HISTORY

**N. KEHSENI
MARKBRON**

Introduction: Understanding Diabetes

Origin and History

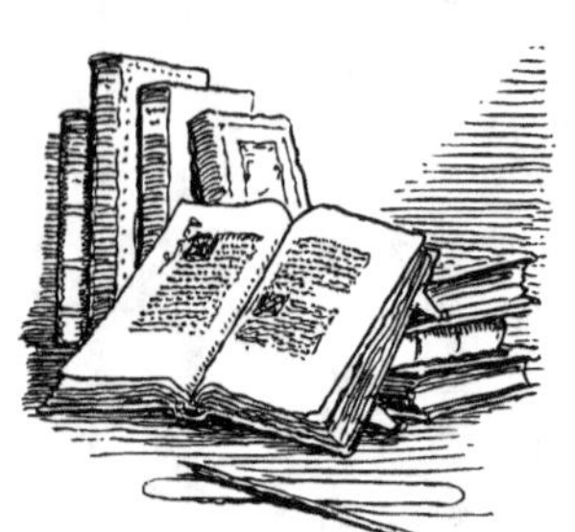

Diabetes is a disease that humans have known about for thousands of years. The onset of diabetes is a complex subject that has been studied by scientists and experts for years. Over the ages, many scientists and experts have studied diabetes, leading to a better understanding of the disease and improved medicines.

The oldest recorded mentions of diabetes were in ancient Egypt. The Ebers Papyrus, an ancient Egyptian medical record dating back to 1500 BC, includes accounts of patients suffering from excessive thirst and profuse urine, which are now known as standard signs of diabetes. These patients were treated with a range of plant-based medicines, including products of fenugreek, which has been found to have antidiabetic qualities.

The unique traits of diabetes, as mentioned in the Ebers Papyrus, include polyuria (excessive urination), polydipsia (excessive thirst), and polyphagia (excessive hunger). Other signs may include weight loss, tiredness, and decreased eyesight. These symptoms are caused by the body's inability to properly control blood sugar levels, which can lead to high amounts of glucose in the blood.

The treatment methods suggested in the Ebers Papyrus for treating diabetes included a variety of plant-based medicines, some of which are still used today. Fenugreek, for example, has been found to help control blood sugar levels and improve insulin sensitivity. Other cures listed in the papyrus include aloe vera, myrrh, and ginger. These plants were used to make poultices, ointments, and drinks that were given directly or consumed. Although the ancient Egyptians had a clear understanding of the signs of diabetes and how to fix them, they did not have the scientific knowledge to explain the root causes of the disease.

In the 5th century BC, Sushruta, a famous Indian surgeon, identified diabetes in his work, "Samhita" (an old Sanskrit text on medicine and surgery). He used the term "madhumeha" to describe the disease, which is marked by pee that is pleasant in taste, sticky to touch, and draws insects (ants). Sushruta also noticed that diabetes was more common among the wealthy classes and linked it to increased consumption of rice, grains, and sweets.

In ancient China, Chang Chung-Ching, known as "the Chinese Hippocrates," identified polyuria, polydipsia, and weight loss as signs of a specific disease around 160–219 AD. Similarly, in the 7th century AD, Chen Chuan reported fragrant urine as a typical sign of diabetes mellitus and named the disease **Hsiao kho-ping**. He noticed other signs, such as intense thirst, copious drinking, and large quantities of sweet-tasting urine. Chen Chuan's partner, Li Hsuan, offered abstention from wine, salt, and intercourse as a possible solution for the sickness. These old Chinese doctors made important advances in early diabetes research and treatment.

Starting in the 8th century, doctors began to discover a link between diabetes and the growth of skin diseases such as furuncles and rat sores. They also found that diabetic people were more sensitive to eye problems. These early findings helped to further understand the general nature of diabetes and its effect on different areas of the body. As research and medical knowledge improved over time, these findings contributed to the development of more effective treatments and control methods for diabetes and its complications.

In the 11th century AD, the Arabo-Islamic physician Avicenna gave a full description of diabetes in his work El-Kanun (Canon of Medicine). Avicenna described diabetes as a chronic disease marked by extreme thirst, frequent urination, and sweet-tasting pee. He understood that diabetes was a result of the body's failure to properly process food and control glucose levels. Avicenna also noticed that the disease was more common among the elderly and those who led a sedentary lifestyle. In addition to outlining the standard signs of diabetes, Avicenna also noticed several problems that could arise from the disease. He noticed that diabetes could add to nerve damage, erectile dysfunction, and gangrene, a situation where tissue death happens due to a lack of blood flow. Avicenna also noted the connection between diabetes and weight loss, which he thought was due to the body's failure to properly utilize nutrients from a meal.

We can see that there is a connection between the different findings made from 1500 BC to the 11th century AD, but there is no suitable scientific understanding to explain the root causes of the disease. But in the 2nd century AD, Aretaeus, probably the best physician of the Greco-Roman period after Hippocrates created the first exact description of diabetes, Aretaeus' correct clinical presentation and understanding of diabetes in the 2nd century AD are remarkable. He described diabetes as a unique and rare disease that affects the kidneys and bladder. The patients suffer from a constant and uncontrolled flow of urine, which is followed by burning thirst and excessive drinking that does not match the amount of urine created. Aretaeus noticed that the disease is ongoing and takes a long time to form, but patients are short-lived once the illness completely takes hold. He described life with diabetes as unpleasant and painful, with symptoms such as vertigo, nervousness, and a burning thirst that cannot be filled. If patients stop drinking, their mouths become dried and dehydrated, and they finally die. Aretaeus suggested that the disease also affects the bowels, causing emaciation, a smaller belly, and visible veins. He proposed a treatment plan that included the consumption of cereals, milk, and wine, as well as the use of cataplasms and Theriac, a famous antiquity cure. Despite his exact clinical account, it remains a mystery how Aretaeus was able to record such a rare disease during a time when scientific understanding and technology were limited just by sight.

In the 17th century, English physician Thomas Willis (1621–1675) used the name "diabetes" to describe the increased urination and thirst associated with the disease, which he thought was caused by the kidneys releasing extra water. The word "mellitus" was later added to describe the sugary taste of the urine, which is caused by the presence of glucose. The name "mellitus" is taken from the Latin word for honey, "mel." Thus, "diabetes mellitus" translates to "sweet siphon" or "sweet flow," in reference to the extra drainage and sweetness of the urine. The term "diabetes mellitus" therefore takes its origin from the work of English surgeon Thomas Willis (1621–1675). In his 1674 book

Pharmaceutice rationalis sive diatriba de medicamentorum operationibus in humano corpore" (Rational Pharmacology or Treatise on the Operations of Medicines in the Human Body), he coined the term "diabetes mellitus," and it continues to be used to describe the metabolic disorder characterized by high blood sugar levels due to insufficient insulin production or resistance to insulin.

An important event in the history of diabetes mellitus happened in 1889, two German physicians, Oscar Minkowski and Von Mering. Prior to their first meeting, von Mering had already discovered in 1886 that phlorizin, a glucoside, could cause brief glucuresis. In 1889, von Mering was conducting studies at the Hoppe Seyler's Institute, based at the University of Strasbourg, while Minkowski was working as an assistant to Professor Bernard Naunyn, a major diabetes expert in Germany. During this period, Minkowski visited Hoppe Seyler's institute to read some chemistry books from the library. By chance, he and Mering had a talk about lipanin, an oil that von Mering used to give to patients with stomach problems. Minkowski disagreed with using lipanin.

This led to a talk on the pancreas's role in the breakdown and absorption of fats. After the conversation, they decided to perform a pancreatectomy on a dog in Naunyn's laboratory that same evening. After the operation, the animal survived and was watched closely by Minkowski, while von Mering had to leave immediately for Colmar due to a family issue. The dog experienced polyuria (increased urination) shortly after the treatment, and when checking its pee, Minkowski found that it contained 12% sugar. At first, Minkowski thought that the dog's diabetes was caused by von Mering's continued use of phlorizin.

As a result, he performed the pancreatectomy on three

additional dogs that had no sugar in their pee prior to the operation, and all three developed glycosuria. Additionally, Minkowski inserted a small piece of pancreas subcutaneously in dogs that had received a pancreatectomy and found that hyperglycemia was avoided until the implant was removed or naturally decayed. Through their trial, Minkowski and von Mering showed that the pancreas is a vital structure of internal release responsible for maintaining glucose balance.

These results were groundbreaking and paved the way for further study into the causes and cures of diabetes. They equally paved the way for Frederick Banting and Charles Best, two Renoun Canadian physicians, to perform their tests on isolating insulin effectively.

In 1923, Frederick Banting and John MacLeod were given the Nobel Prize in Medicine for their discovery of insulin, which was a great success that led to a major scientific debate. Frederick Banting, a young Canadian surgeon, was allowed into the laboratory of Professor John Macleod, a famous scientist at the University of Toronto who had a keen interest in diabetes. In 1920, Moses Barron, a physician from Minnesota, wrote a paper about the islets of Langerhans and their connection to diabetes. He stated that continuing Minkowski and von Mering's studies could lead to the discovery of a drug to control diabetes. After being inspired by Barron's piece, Frederick Banting turned his attention towards studying diabetes.

At that time, the famous English scientist Ernest Starling (1886–1927) made a statement: "We don't know yet how the pancreas affects sugar production or utilization in the same animal. It is usually believed that it secretes into the bloodstream a hormone that may pass to the tissues and allow them to utilize sugar or pass to the liver and block the sugar production of this organ. We have been unable to imitate the action of the pancreas, still in arterial link with the body, by injection or administration of the samples of this organ."

Beginning on May 16, 1921, Frederick Banting started working together with a young medical student named Charles Best. They performed tests on dogs, initially ligating the pancreatic tubes, which resulted in the shortening of the exocrine area.

Nearly ten weeks later, they took the degenerated liver from the dog. They then proceeded to crush the atrophied pancreatic glands in a cool mill and freeze them in salt water. The mass was then ground down and added to 100 mL of physiological salt. They then administered 5 mL of this extract intravenously to a dog whose pancreas had been removed.

Within two hours, the dog's blood sugar had greatly dropped. They performed the experiment several times on other diabetic dogs, getting similar findings. They also worked with the fetal calf pancreas and used different methods of administration, such as intramuscular and oral.

At the end of 1921, James Collip, a skilled scientist, joined the team and developed a better extraction and filtering method. The drug they got was originally called "insletin" by the team, but was later named "insulin" by MacLeod. The next step was to test insulin on people.

On January 11, 1922, they gave insulin to Leonard Thompson, a 14-year-old boy with diabetes who was being treated at Toronto Hospital. Thompson was also following a strict fasting diet suggested by Frederick Madison Allen (1879–1964) and was in serious condition. He got 15 mL of insulin shot into his thigh, but he developed abscesses at the injection site and became even sicker.

Collip made further changes to the quality of insulin, and on January 23, Thompson got a second shot, which produced great results. In just 24 hours, his blood glucose levels dropped from 520 mg/dL to 120 mg/dL, and his urine ketones vanished. Thompson continued to receive care with insulin and lived for another 13 years before passing away from pneumonia at the age of 27.

In 1923, the Nobel Committee made the decision to award Frederick Banting and MacLeod for the discovery of insulin. Frederick Banting was extremely upset because he thought that Charles Best should share the prize with him instead of MacLeod. As a result, he chose to share his cash gift with Charles Best. In turn, MacLeod shared his award with Collip.
A critical milestone in the history of diabetes was achieved, setting the way for future improvements. Insulin processing methods continued to improve, and new insulin formulations were developed.

In the following years, scientists made important findings in the area of diabetes studies. In 1955, Nobel Prize winner Fred Sanger (1918–2013) outlined the structure of insulin. In 1967, Donald Steiner (1930–2014) and his colleagues found proinsulin and developed the radioimmunoassay for C-peptide, which is still used today to measure endogenous insulin release. That same year, the first pancreas replacement in a person was performed by William Kelly, Richard Lillehei (1927–1981), and their team at the University of Minnesota. In 1972, the U100 insulin was launched to improve dosing efficiency. In 1982, recombinant human insulin became available, and in the early 1990s, insulin pen delivery devices gained favor. This was followed by the finding of short-acting insulin analogs in 1996 and long-acting insulin analogs in 2001.

What is Diabetes?

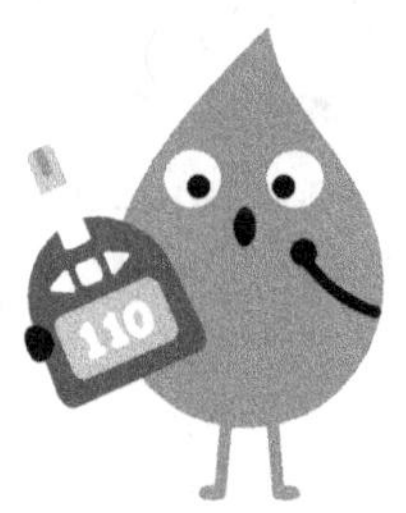

Diabetes, often referred to as diabetes mellitus, is a chronic medical condition that affects how the body manages blood sugar (glucose) levels. When a person's pancreas, an organ that plays a crucial role in both digestion and regulating the amount of glucose in the blood, produces insufficient insulin, or when the body cannot effectively use the insulin produced by the pancreas, it causes glucose to stockpile in the blood. This accumulation of glucose in the blood over a long period result in a medical condition known as diabetes.

Note:

We have to keep in mind that anytime we talk of sugar or blood sugar, we're referring to glucose.

The word "glucose" originates from the Greek term for "sweet." It represents a form of sugar obtained from the food we consume, serving as a source of energy for the body. When glucose circulates through the bloodstream, it is referred to as blood glucose or blood sugar.

In order to have a clear and concise understanding of diabetes in a straightforward and efficient manner, it is crucial to have a grasp of certain bodily processes. Below are some definitions of biological terms that will facilitate our understanding of diabetes.

The Cells

A cell is the basic structural and functional unit of all living organisms.

It is the smallest independently functioning unit of life and can perform a variety of vital functions within an organism. Cells are the building blocks of tissues, organs, and ultimately, the entire organism.

Each cell has certain receptors on its surface. These receptors can have a certain number of functions. Some of which are: signal detection, signal transduction, cellular response, cell communication, and regulation of biological processes.

Glucose

When we eat foods rich in carbohydrates, protein, vitamins, fats, and other nutrients, our digestive system breaks down these nutrients into their basic components. Glucose is derived from foods rich in carbohydrates. When carbohydrate-rich meals get into the digestive system, they are broken down into smaller molecules, such as glucose. Carbohydrates are a compact form of nutrients consisting of two or more smaller nutrients, such as glucose, fructose, and galactose.

Glucose is a type of sugar, often referred to as a simple sugar or monosaccharide. It is a fundamental and essential source of energy for living organisms, including humans. Glucose is obtained primarily from the digestion of carbohydrates in foods like bread, pasta, fruits, and vegetables. During digestion, carbohydrates are broken down into glucose, which is then absorbed into the bloodstream. This circulating glucose serves as a vital fuel for cells, tissues, and organs, providing the energy necessary for various bodily functions and physical activities.

The Pancreas 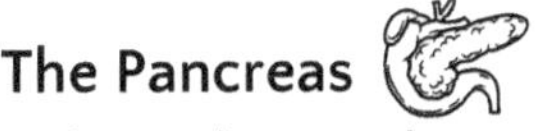

When glucose leaves the digestive system and is absorbed

into the blood stream, a certain organ known as the pancreas detects the presence of glucose in the blood. The pancreas is located in the abdomen, behind the stomach, and deep within the upper part of the abdomen. It is positioned horizontally, behind and slightly below the lower part of the ribcage. The pancreas is relatively flat and elongated, with one end connected to the duodenum (the first part of the small intestine) and the other end extending towards the spleen. The pancreas has several functions, some of which are:

The pancreas has several functions, some of which are:
- Regulation of blood sugar levels
- Secretion of digestive enzymes into the small intestine to aid in the digestion of carbohydrates, proteins, and fats
- Production of bicarbonate, a substance that helps neutralize stomach acid as food enters the small intestine.

There is a specialized group of cells located in the pancreas called "beta cells." These cells are part of the pancreatic islets (or islets of Langerhans) and play a crucial role in regulating blood glucose levels.

Note:

The "islets of Langerhans" are clusters of specialized cells found within the pancreas. These islets are named after the German pathologist Paul Langerhans, who first described them in the 19th century.

*The islets of Langerhans have two main types of cells with distinct functions: **alpha** and **beta** cells*

.

Here's how the pancreas detects the presence of glucose and maintains blood sugar balance:

- **Sensing Blood Glucose Levels:** Beta cells in the pancreas have glucose receptors on their surface. These receptors are sensitive to changes in blood glucose levels.
- **Release of Insulin:** When blood glucose levels rise, such as after eating a meal rich in carbohydrate, the beta cells detect the increase in blood sugar. In response, they release the hormone insulin into the bloodstream, which helps lower blood sugar levels when they are too high.

The islets of Langerhans are crucial for maintaining blood glucose homeostasis, as they control the release of insulin and **glucagon** in response to changes in blood sugar levels. Dysfunction in these islets can lead to disorders like diabetes mellitus, which is characterized by impaired blood sugar regulation.

Insulin

This is the hormone secreted by the beta cells of the pancreas in response to high levels of glucose in the blood. It is important to remember this hormone and its function because it will go a long way in our study of diabetes.

A Simple Explanation of How Insulin Works:

When beta cells secrete insulin into the blood stream in response to a high glucose level, it travels around the body in order to reduce blood glucose (sugar) levels. It does this by ushering the glucose into the cells, where it will be used for energy. You can think of insulin as a key that opens up the cell for glucose to be able to go in. Without insulin, glucose will be unable to enter the cells, and as a result, it will just float around the body. Below is a more detailed explanation of how insulin works.

- **After Eating:** When we eat, the carbohydrates in our food are digested and broken down into glucose, which enters our bloodstream, causing our blood sugar levels to rise.
- **Insulin Release:** When blood sugar rises, the pancreas releases insulin into the bloodstream.
- **Unlocking Cells:** Insulin acts like a key that fits into special receptors on the surface of our cells. When insulin binds to these receptors, it signals the cell to open up.
- **Glucose Entry:** With the cell doors open, glucose can now enter the cells. Once inside, glucose is used by the cells for energy production, and the energy produced enables us to carry out our daily activities like walking, talking, and even eating.
- **Lowering Blood Sugar:** As glucose enters the cells, the amount of glucose in the bloodstream decreases. This helps lower blood sugar levels and keeps them within a healthy range.

Diabetes comes in three basic forms: type 1, type 2, and gestational diabetes. We will look at type 1 and gestational diabetes in this chapter and focus extensively on type 2 diabetes in the next chapter.

Types of Diabetes

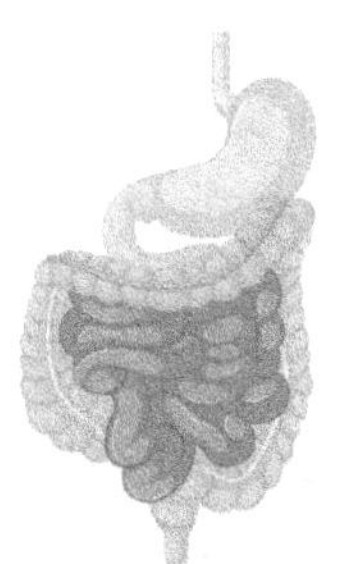

Type 1 diabetes

In the previous paragraphs, we talked about the pancreas as an organ that regulates blood sugar levels by producing a hormone called insulin. In type 1 diabetes, the body's immune system mistakenly attacks and destroys the beta cells in the pancreas, which are responsible for producing insulin. This will result in very little or no insulin production by the pancreas and consequently lead to high blood sugar levels (hyperglycemia), which are the main criteria for diagnosing diabetes. This autoimmune destruction of pancreatic beta cells leads to type 1 diabetes.

The science behind the destruction of the pancreatic beta cells by the immune system is a very complex mechanism, but let's put it in simple terms.
This autoimmune response (the body attacking itself by mistake) is caused by a combination of genetic and environmental factors. The immune system is like an army of soldiers that helps the body fight off harmful organisms and pathogens like germs that can make you sick. But sometimes, the immune system gets confused and thinks that healthy cells in the body are actually bad guys that need to be attacked.

In type 1 diabetes, the immune system mistakenly identifies the beta cells in the pancreas as invaders and attacks them. It is important to note that beta cells are special cells in the pancreas that secrete a hormone called insulin, which helps the body use sugar from the food we eat for energy production in the cell. Without enough insulin, the sugar builds up in the blood and can't be used by the body's cells for daily metabolic processes.

The attack on the beta cells is carried out by a type of immune cell called T cells. These T cells recognize specific proteins called peptides that are found on the surface of the beta cells. In a type 1 diabetes patient, these T cells recognize these peptides as foreign, and they start attacking the beta cells. Over time, more and more beta cells are destroyed, and the pancreas can't produce enough insulin to channel glucose into the cells, which leads to high blood sugar levels and eventually causes type 1 diabetes.

Type 1 diabetes can develop at any age, but it is most commonly diagnosed in children, adolescents, and young adults. In fact, it used to be known as **"juvenile diabetes"** because of its prevalence in young people.

According to the American Diabetes Association (ADA), about 2 million Americans have Type 1 diabetes, and it accounts for approximately 5-10% of all diagnosed cases of diabetes in the United States. The peak age of onset for Type 1 diabetes is between 10 and 14 years old, although it can occur at any age, from infancy to adulthood.

Note: *T-cells: T-cells, also known as T lymphocytes, are a type of white blood cell that plays a critical role in the immune system's defense against infections and diseases. They are one of the two main types of lymphocytes, with the other being B-cells.*

Here are some key characteristics and functions of T-cells:

- *Cell-Mediated Immunity: T-cells are primarily responsible for cell-mediated immunity, which means they directly attack and destroy infected or abnormal cells in the body. This is particularly important in fighting viral infections and combating cancerous cells.*

- *Antigen Recognition: T-cells recognize specific molecules called antigens, which are typically present on the surface of infected cells or pathogens (such as viruses or bacteria). T-cell receptors (TCRs) on the surface of T-cells bind to these antigens, allowing T-cells to identify the threat.*

Signs and Symptoms of Type 1 Diabetes

Type 1 diabetes can present with various signs and symptoms, which are often noticeable and may develop relatively quickly. Common signs and symptoms of type 1 diabetes include:

- Excessive Thirst (Polydipsia): People with type 1 diabetes often experience extreme thirst, as the high blood sugar levels lead to increased urine production, causing dehydration.
- Frequent Urination (Polyuria): Increased glucose levels in the blood can lead to frequent urination as the body attempts to eliminate excess sugar through urine.
- Unexplained Weight Loss: Despite increased hunger and food intake, individuals with type 1 diabetes may lose weight unintentionally. This is because the body cannot use glucose for energy effectively, so it breaks down stored fat and muscle tissue for energy.
- Extreme Hunger (Polyphagia): Increased appetite and persistent hunger are common symptoms, as cells are deprived

of glucose even though it is abundant in the bloodstream.

- Fatigue and Weakness: Insufficient glucose uptake by cells leads to reduced energy production by these cells and can result in fatigue and weakness, making it difficult to carry out daily activities.
- Blurred Vision: High blood sugar levels can affect the lenses of the eyes, leading to temporary changes in vision, such as blurriness.
- Irritability: Mood swings, irritability, and changes in behavior are sometimes observed, particularly in children and adolescents.
- Frequent Infections: Individuals with untreated type 1 diabetes may be more susceptible to infections, as high blood sugar levels can weaken the immune system
- Ketoacidosis (in severe cases): If type 1 diabetes is left untreated or poorly managed, it can lead to a life-threatening condition called diabetic ketoacidosis (DKA). Symptoms of DKA include nausea, vomiting, abdominal pain, fruity-scented breath, and confusion.

Risk Factors for Type 1 Diabetes

Numerous factors exist that can contribute to the development of type 1 diabetes. However, let us examine the key risk factors.

• Genetics and Family History

If someone in your family has type 1 diabetes, it can increase your chances of developing it too. For example, if your mother or father has type 1 diabetes, your risk is higher. The risk is equally higher for siblings, especially if they were diagnosed at a young age. In fact, for identical twins, the risk of the other twin developing type 1 diabetes is as high as 1 in 3. For parents of patients with type 1 diabetes, the risk of developing diabetes by the age of 40 is about 2.6%, and it's higher for fathers compared to mothers. By the age of 60, around 10% of close relatives may develop type 1 diabetes. However, it's important to note that these familial cases account for less than 10% of all type 1 diabetes cases, and they don't differ from cases that occur randomly in terms of certain genetic factors or the presence of autoantibodies.

The increased risk of developing type 1 diabetes in family members is due to a combination of shared genes and a shared environment. The genes most strongly associated with type 1 diabetes are certain versions of the **HLA class II genes**. These genes account for about 30% to 50% of the genetic risk for the disease. There are over 50 other genetic regions, apart from HLA, that have been identified as contributing to the risk of type 1 diabetes, but each of these regions has a smaller effect on the overall risk. Some of the non-HLA genes that have been studied include **INS** and **PTPN22**. However, these genes alone may not have a significant impact on developing the disease. They might need to work together with other factors, such as environmental exposures, for the disease to occur (known as gene-environment interaction).

Note:

1. *Human leukocyte antigen (HLA) class II genes*

HLA class II genes are like instruction manuals in our DNA that help our immune system recognize and respond to invaders like germs. These genes create proteins called HLA class II molecules, which reveal parts of these invaders to our immune cells. This helps our immune system figure out how to fight off the pathogens and keep us healthy. HLA class II genes are important for our body's defense against infections and diseases

2. ***INS (Insulin Gene):***

The INS gene is responsible for producing the hormone insulin. Mutations or variations in the INS gene can affect insulin production and contribute to conditions like diabetes.

3. ***PTPN22 (Protein Tyrosine Phosphatase Non-Receptor Type 22):***

PTPN22 is a gene that codes for a protein involved in regulating immune responses. Specifically, it produces a protein that helps control the activation of immune cells called T cells. T-cells play a vital role in the immune system's response to infections and the recognition of self from non-self (such as distinguishing between healthy cells and invading pathogens). Variations in the PTPN22 gene have been associated with an increased risk of autoimmune diseases, where the immune system mistakenly attacks the body's own tissues. These conditions include rheumatoid arthritis, type 1 diabetes, and others. PTPN22 gene variants can influence the balance of immune responses, making individuals more susceptible to autoimmune disorders.

• Viral Infections

Sometimes, certain viruses can play a role in causing type 1 diabetes, although it is challenging to provide definitive proof. The signs of viral infections that may contribute to the development of diabetes in the future can be difficult to detect because there is usually a long time between the infection and the actual onset of diabetes. Researchers have identified several potential viral triggers, and the most promising leads are discussed here.

One group of viruses called enteroviruses has shown associations with type 1 diabetes in studies conducted on both animals and humans. These viruses have a particular affinity for the cells in the pancreas that produce insulin (beta cells).

They have been found in the pancreas of individuals with type 1 diabetes. Studies on animals suggest that the timing of the infection may be crucial. The outcome of the infection can vary between individuals who already have autoimmune activity against their pancreatic cells and those whose cells are not affected. The outcome is also influenced by complex interactions between the virus and the body's immune system. Variations in specific genes related to the immune system can determine the severity of a viral infection.

Despite many studies conducted using different approaches, the relationship between enteroviruses and type 1 diabetes remains controversial. In most cases, the diagnosis of type 1 diabetes comes after a long period of preclinical autoimmune activity against the pancreas. The viruses present at the time of diagnosis may have infected the individual late in the disease process, rather than triggering it. Alternatively, the triggering infection may have already been cleared from the body by the time of diagnosis, unless the virus is able to persist in the body. Enterovirus infections might potentially initiate autoimmune activity against the pancreas, influence the progression towards clinical type 1 diabetes, or both.

Note: *Enteroviruses are a group of viruses belonging to the Picornaviridae family. These viruses are named for their ability to enter the human body through the digestive tract (entero means "intestine"). Enteroviruses are a common cause of various infections, including mild illnesses like the common cold as well as more severe conditions such as viral meningitis and myocarditis (inflammation of the heart muscle).*

• Food and Seasonal Changes

Children are more likely to develop type 1 diabetes in the autumn and winter months, while the risk is lower in the spring and summer. This pattern is observed in both the northern and southern hemispheres, similar to the seasonality of viral infections. However, there is a more noticeable seasonal variation in children between the ages of 11 and 15 compared to those diagnosed before the age of 5. This could be because older children are more likely to be in school, making it easier to detect the signs and symptoms of diabetes. The development of islet autoimmunity, which is associated with type 1 diabetes, may also be influenced by environmental factors during pregnancy. This is suggested by the presence of *islet autoantibodies* in cord blood, which show a seasonal pattern, as well as the seasonal distribution of birth dates among type 1 diabetes patients.

During the first year of a baby's life, they are introduced to different types of food in addition to breast milk substitutes like infant formulas. These foods can affect the baby's immune system and their risk of developing certain autoimmune conditions, such as type 1 diabetes.

Several studies have looked at when specific foods are introduced to babies and how it relates to their risk of developing islet autoimmunity, which is associated with type 1 diabetes. For example, one study found that introducing cereals before the baby is three months old increases the risk, while introducing them between four and six months seems to have a protective effect. However, different studies have produced conflicting results about whether *gluten*, a component of cereals, is the main driving factor behind this increased risk.

Another study from Finland discovered that introducing gluten-containing cereals between 5 and 5.5 months of age increases the risk of islet autoimmunity, but only during the first three years

Introducing gluten earlier than five months does not seem to increase the risk.

Gluten has been extensively studied because it is also the trigger for celiac disease, another autoimmune condition similar to type 1 diabetes. Researchers found that gluten can trigger the onset of islet autoimmunity in diabetes-prone rats. They also identified a wheat protein called Glb1 that may be associated with damaging the cells responsible for insulin production. Some studies showed that a gluten-free diet may improve the function of these cells in children with islet autoantibodies.

However, a study found that delayed gluten exposure until the baby was 12 months old did not significantly reduce the risk of islet autoimmunity in genetically at-risk children, nor did it increase the risk.

In addition to gluten and cereals, other solid foods in the baby's diet have also been linked to an increased risk of islet autoimmunity. For example, introducing root vegetables before four months of age and eggs before eight months increased the risk during the first three years of life.

The differences in findings across studies may be due to variations in the first solid foods typically introduced to babies in different countries. For example, in the United States, cereals, particularly rice cereal, are often the first solids introduced, while in other countries, root vegetables and fruits are more common.

Recent studies have also looked at how these dietary exposures relate to the development of clinical diabetes in children at risk for type 1 diabetes. Both early and late introductions of solid foods were found to predict the development of type 1 diabetes. Early exposure to fruit and late exposure to rice or oats specifically predicted type 1 diabetes. Delaying gluten-containing foods until after six months did not increase the risk of islet autoimmunity or type 1 diabetes.

Overall, these studies suggest that there are specific times during infancy when introducing certain foods may increase the risk of developing islet autoimmunity and type 1 diabetes. The timing of exposure may be related to the baby's immune response and the maturity of their gut immune system. Early exposure might trigger an abnormal immune response to the foods in susceptible individuals, while late exposure could be influenced by larger food amounts given to older children, nutrient deficiencies, or stopping breastfeeding before introducing solid foods, which removes the protective effects of breast milk.

Note:

1. *Gluten: Gluten is a protein found in certain grains, most notably wheat, barley, rye, and their derivatives. It is composed of two main proteins: gliadin and glutenin. Gluten provides elasticity and structure to dough, making it a crucial component in many baked goods.*

2. *Autoimmunity: Autoimmunity is a condition in which the immune system mistakenly targets and attacks the body's own tissues and cells. In a healthy immune system, the body can distinguish between its own cells and foreign invaders (such as viruses or bacteria). However, in cases of autoimmunity, the immune system loses this ability to differentiate and starts attacking normal, healthy tissues as if they were foreign invaders.*

Autoimmune diseases can affect various parts of the body and result in a wide range of symptoms and health problems. Some common autoimmune diseases include rheumatoid arthritis, systemic lupus erythematosus, type 1 diabetes, multiple sclerosis, and celiac disease, among others.

Complications of Type 1 Diabetes Diabetic ketoacidosis (DKA)

Diabetic ketoacidosis (DKA) is a severe and potentially life-threatening complication that can occur when an individual has type 1 diabetes. Diabetic ketoacidosis is a condition wherein the blood becomes acidic due to the presence of ketone bodies. DKA is mostly associated with type 1 diabetes, but type 2 diabetics are also susceptible. In this section, we will try to explain how diabetic ketoacidosis comes about in type 1 diabetes patients and all the processes that cause this disease to be so deadly. In order to have a full grasp of what diabetic ketoacidosis is and how it affects the body, it is important to understand the processes by which the body manages glucose.

The Genesis of Diabetic Ketoacidosis

One pretty interesting thing about our body is that it is able to maintain a constant range of blood glucose, about 60 to 150 milligrams of glucose per deciliter of blood (3.33 to 8.33 millimoles of glucose per liter of blood.). The reason why the body keeps the blood glucose at a constant level is because some very important organs and tissues in our body, such as the brain, the kidney, and the eyes, rely heavily on glucose for the production of energy, and equally because high levels of glucose tend to damage the blood vessels; therefore, a dysregulation in the levels of glucose could have detrimental effects on these organs and your blood vessels.

The body maintains constant glucose levels through a complex and tightly regulated process known as *glucose homeostasis.* This involves the coordination of various organs, hormones, and physiological mechanisms to ensure that blood glucose levels remain within a narrow range. The key players in glucose homeostasis include insulin, glucagon, the liver, muscles, and adipose tissue.

Note

Glucagon: *Glucagon is a hormone produced by the alpha cells of the pancreas. They help raise blood sugar levels. It's the opposite of insulin. It does so by stimulating the liver to convert stored **glycogen** into glucose, which is then released into the bloodstream. This process is important for maintaining a stable level of glucose in the body, especially during periods of fasting or between meals.*

Glycogen: *Glycogen is a long chain of glucose molecules linked together. It is a stored form of glucose that the body converts when there is excess glucose in the blood. When the body needs energy between meals or during physical activity, it can quickly break down glycogen back into glucose and release it into the bloodstream. This glucose can then be used by cells for energy production*

We know that in type 1 diabetes, there is destruction of the beta cells, which are responsible for the secretion of insulin, and as we have seen above, insulin is one of the hormones responsible for glucose homeostasis. Another interesting thing to note in type 1 diabetes is that the autoimmune destruction of pancreatic cells may not be limited to beta cells. Other cells within the pancreas, such as alpha cells (which produce glucagon), may also be affected to some extent. However, the primary target and the most severe damage occur in the beta cells.

As these cells responsible for the secretion of hormones that play a major role in glucose homeostasis get destroyed, the body loses the ability to keep blood glucose levels normal. This may result in dysregulation of blood sugar levels, and as such, an individual suffering from type 1 diabetes may experience hypoglycemia (low blood glucose) as well as hyperglycemia (high blood glucose) because cells of the organ responsible for glucose homeostasis are destroyed.

Now, at this point, it is no surprise that in type 1 diabetes, there is destruction of the beta cells responsible for producing insulin, leading to insulin deficiency and eventually resulting in little or no glucose getting into the cells. When this happens, the brain is triggered to think that the reason why glucose isn't getting into the cell is due to the fact that the individual has not eaten a glucose-rich meal. It is important to remember that the reason the brain thinks this way is because the organ (pancreas) that detects high blood glucose and regulates the blood sugar level is destroyed, and as such, the brain isn't able to detect if the blood glucose is high or low. The only way for the brain to tell if the blood glucose is high will depend on how the cells react by either opening up for glucose to go in, signifying high glucose, or not opening, signifying low or no glucose. In this case, since the cells cannot take up glucose due to the lack of insulin, the brain will be triggered to think that the individual has not eaten and will then activate various metabolic processes that will increase the amount of glucose in the blood. Note here that there is already glucose present in the blood, but the brain has lost its ability to detect how high or low blood glucose levels are due to the destruction of the pancreas by the immune system.

Another fascinating aspect of the body is its ability to produce glucose on its own.

It basically just takes some protein molecules lying around and joins them through a series of processes to form glucose. Below are some processes the body will use to increase the amount of glucose in the body.

- Glycogenolysis

Anytime you eat a meal rich in carbohydrates, your blood glucose goes up. Now, the body, through a special storage mechanism, transforms the excess glucose into **glycogen** in the liver and stores it in your skeletal muscles and in the liver itself. You can think of **glycogen** as multiple glucose molecules linked together, creating a compact and easy to store form of glucose. Now, when the body needs to carry out a physical activity that requires some level of energy, such as running or playing, signals are sent to initiate the process of glycogenolysis. In simple terms, this is just the body breaking down glycogen (a compact form of glucose adequate for storage) back into glucose and supplying it to the cells in order to perform the task at hand.

2.Gluconeogenesis

Gluconeogenesis is exactly what the name implies: the creation of new glucose. One very fascinating aspect of the human body is the fact that it is able to create glucose from non-carbohydrate sources. This basically means that our body takes precursor molecules such as protein and lactate and, in a metabolic series of processes, produces glucose, which will eventually be used as fuel for the cells.

When these processes mentioned above (glycogenolysis and gluconeogenesis) occur, they just go to increase the amount of glucose in the blood as the brain thinks that the individual lacks glucose, causing a more and more hyperglycemic state. As all of this glucose circulates in the body, the excess of it is excreted as urine.

This excess urination causes increased thirst and dehydration, all of which are typical symptoms of type 1 diabetes. Over time, the brain will notice that the glucose being produced by the processes of glucose formation listed above does not solve the problem of reduced energy production by the cell. So what does it do?

The brain then shifts to an alternative source of energy production since the cell doesn't respond to glucose to produce energy. The body, through the process of **lipolysis,** will break down fats from fat stores (adipose tissues), and these broken-down fat cells will travel to the liver to undergo a metabolic process called **ketogenesis**, which is the production of ketone bodies through the breakdown of fats and some proteins. Now, the body uses these ketones as an alternative source of energy. It is important to note that ketogenesis is a natural metabolic process that can occur in the body, and it mostly occurs when our body is in a fasting state, but in the case of DKA, the body will have no choice but to activate this mechanism.

As more and more ketones are produced through the breakdown of fat molecules, very large amounts of ketones accumulate in the blood, a condition known as **ketonemia**. Ketonemia eventually leads to **ketonuria**, which is the excretion of ketones in urine, and severe weight loss as the fats in the muscles are being broken down to produce energy.

One thing about ketones is that they are acidic compounds, and when they accumulate in the blood, they can alter the **blood's PH** and lead to a condition called **metabolic acidosis.** This is a disruption in the body's acid-base balance, shifting it towards acidity. This acidic nature of the blood damages a lot of enzymes, hormones, and some of the most vital organs in the body.

Now, a combination of hyperglycemia, insulin deficiency, ketogenesis resulting in ketonemia, and metabolic acidosis is what we refer to as diabetic ketoacidosis.

Note

Lipolisis: *Lipolysis is the process by which fats (lipids) are broken down in the body to release fatty acids. This process typically occurs in fat cells (adipocytes) and is activated during periods of fasting, exercise, or when the body needs additional energy. The released fatty acids can then be used by the body as a source of energy.*

Ketogenesis: *Ketogenesis is the process in which the body produces ketone bodies, such as beta-hydroxybutyrate, as a result of breaking down fats for energy when glucose is scarce, such as during fasting or on a low-carbohydrate diet.*

Ketones: *Ketones, or ketone bodies, are molecules produced from fatty acids during periods of low food intake (fasting), carbohydrate restrictive diets, prolonged intense exercise, or untreated type 1 diabetes. They serve as an alternative energy source for the body, particularly for the brain, when glucose is not readily available.*

Ketonemia: *Ketonemia is simply the presence of ketone bodies in the blood, which typically occurs when the body is burning fat for fuel instead of glucose.*

Ketonuria: *Ketoneuria refers to the presence of ketone bodies in the urine, which can indicate that the body is breaking down fat for energy instead of using glucose.*

Gestational Diabetes 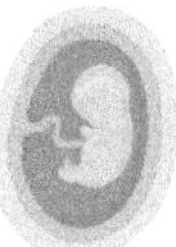

Gestational diabetes mellitus, abbreviated as GDM, is a common condition that occurs during pregnancy and is typically diagnosed around the third trimester. Gestational diabetes shares similarities with type 2 diabetes, as it is characterized by elevated blood sugar levels (hyperglycemia) and issues with insulin resistance.

Normal Pregnancy and Pancreatic Function:

To ensure normal fetal growth during pregnancy, the body of a pregnant woman undergoes some physiological changes to make sure that the fetus consistently receives an adequate supply of glucose. Some of these changes include:

1. **Decreased Maternal Insulin Sensitivity**: During pregnancy, maternal tissues become less sensitive to the action of insulin. This reduced sensitivity means that the effects of insulin on maternal tissues are diminished, and as such, less glucose is getting into the cells of the maternal tissues. This happens because the body intends to channel more glucose into the fetus for adequate fetal growth. As a result, more glucose remains in the maternal bloodstream.

2. **Maternal Pancreatic Changes:** Over time, maternal pancreatic cells undergo hyperplasia (an increase in the number of cells in an organ or tissue, in this case the pancreas), due to the decreased insulin sensitivity in maternal tissues. This essentially happens because the body needs more insulin to be able to feed the mother and the baby, and also because the mother's body is trying to overcome the decrease in insulin sensitivity, which is mostly influenced by hormones released by the placenta of the fetus.

3. Insulin Resistance in Gestational Diabetes:

When a pregnant woman has gestational diabetes, there is a more significant decrease in maternal insulin sensitivity. A condition known as insulin resistance. The development of insulin resistance in gestational diabetes is thought to be influenced by factors such as hormones produced by the placenta, ***including growth hormones, CRH (corticotropin-releasing hormone),*** and ***placental lactogen***. These hormones may contribute to decreased insulin sensitivity in maternal tissues, ultimately affecting glucose regulation during pregnancy.

After a GDM mother eats, her blood glucose levels naturally rise, leading to a state of hyperglycemia (elevated blood sugar). In response to hyperglycemia, the pancreas releases insulin into circulation. The released insulin circulates in the maternal bloodstream and targets the target cells responsible for the absorption of glucose, but the increased insulin resistance in GDM prevents the cells from taking up glucose normally, and glucose stockpiles in the bloodstream, leading to hyperglycemia. This hyperglycemia in the maternal circulation also has an impact on the developing fetus. Since there is a very high level of glucose in the mother's blood streams, the high blood glucose in the mother can cross the placenta and enter fetal circulation. This leads to an increase in blood glucose levels in the fetus, causing fetal hyperglycemia. To cope with elevated maternal blood glucose levels, the fetal pancreas produces its own insulin. This additional fetal insulin helps fetal tissues take up the excess glucose available, promoting fetal growth. This increase in glucose absorption in the fetus can result in excessive fetal growth, leading to a larger-than-average baby, a condition known as macrosomia. This is why, most often, pregnant women suffering from GDM give birth through a C-section due to the large size of the baby.

Some symptoms associated with gestational diabetes include:
- Polyuria (increased urination).
- Polyphagia (increased hunger)
- Paresthesia (uncommon but possible tingling sensations)
- Polydipsia (increased thirst)

However, it's important to note that these symptoms are not very specific to gestational diabetes. In fact, gestational diabetes often remains asymptomatic.

Diagnosis of Gestational Diabetes Mellitus

The diagnosis of GDM is typically conducted during routine screening between 24 and 28 weeks. Two common methods are used for diagnosis:

1. **Fasting Blood Glucose Test:** A fasting blood glucose measurement is taken between weeks 24 and 28 of pregnancy. Before the test, the GDM mom is asked to fast for a certain period of time, usually overnight (8 to 12 hours), to ensure accurate results. During this time, they can only drink water and should avoid consuming any food or beverages that could affect blood sugar levels. Once the fasting period is over, a small sample of blood is taken from a vein, usually from the arm, using a needle. This blood sample is collected in a test tube or vial. The blood sample is then sent to a laboratory for analysis. In the lab, technicians measure the concentration of glucose in the blood sample using specialized equipment. A fasting blood glucose level greater than 5.1 millimoles per liter (91.8 milligrams per deciliter.) can indicate the presence of GDM.

2. **Oral Glucose Tolerance Test (OGTT):** This test involves

drinking a sugary solution, followed by blood glucose measurements at specific time intervals (usually one hour and two hours after drinking the solution). A diagnosis of GDM can be made if:

- Blood glucose is greater than 10 millimoles per liter (180 milligrams per deciliter) after one hour.
- Blood glucose is greater than 8.5 millimoles per liter (153 milligrams per deciliter) after two hours.

These values are significant because, in a normal pregnancy, insulin helps to lower blood glucose levels relatively quickly after consuming a glucose-rich solution. However, in the presence of insulin resistance or reduced sensitivity, blood glucose levels take longer to decrease after glucose ingestion, leading to elevated values during the OGTT.

It's worth noting that the criteria for diagnosing GDM during pregnancy are different from those for diagnosing type 2 diabetes in non-pregnant individuals. The diagnostic criteria for type 2 diabetes outside of pregnancy typically include a fasting blood glucose level greater than 7 millimoles per liter (126 milligrams per deciliter) or a random blood glucose level greater than 11 millimoles per liter (198 milligrams per deciliter) with symptoms of diabetes. These criteria are part of what is sometimes referred to as the "seven-eleven" rule for diagnosing type 2 diabetes.

Complications of Gestational Diabetes

The complications of gestational diabetes can be categorized into maternal, fetal, and infant complications:

Maternal Complications of Gestational Diabetes:

- **Hypertensive Disorders:** Women with gestational diabetes may be at an increased risk of developing hypertensive disorders during pregnancy.

Hypertensive disorders in gestational diabetes mellitus (GDM) refer to a group of conditions characterized by high blood pressure that occur during pregnancy in women who also have gestational diabetes. These conditions can include:

1. Gestational hypertension: This is a form of high blood pressure that develops after the 20th week of pregnancy in women who previously had normal blood pressure. It typically resolves after childbirth.
2. Preeclampsia: Preeclampsia is a more serious condition that involves high blood pressure along with damage to organs such as the liver and kidneys. It can lead to complications for both the mother and the baby if not properly managed. Women with GDM are at a higher risk of developing preeclampsia.
3. Eclampsia: Eclampsia is a severe and life-threatening complication of preeclampsia, characterized by seizures in a pregnant woman who has high blood pressure. It requires immediate medical attention.

- **Increased Risk of Infection**: There may be a higher risk of infections and, in some cases, an increased likelihood of requiring a cesarean section (C-section) delivery.
- **Future Risk of Diabetes Type 2**: Having gestational diabetes can elevate the risk of developing type 2 diabetes in the future.
- **Treatment Complications**: Sometimes, the treatment of gestational diabetes, especially if insulin is administered late, can lead to hypoglycemia (low blood sugar) in the mother.

Fetal Complications of Gestational Diabetes:
- **Fetal hyperinsulinemia**: Elevated blood glucose levels in the mother can lead to high levels of glucose in the fetus, which

will result in increased insulin production in the fetus. This results in greater glucose uptake by fetal tissues, causing macrosomia, which means the baby is larger than average.

- **Fetal Hyperglycemia:** When the baby (fetus) inside a pregnant woman has high levels of sugar in her blood, it can lead to a situation where the baby's kidneys start producing more urine. This increased urine production by the baby is known as "fetal osmotic diuresis." Now, this extra urine from the baby doesn't just stay inside the baby's body—it goes into the amniotic fluid surrounding the baby in the womb. Amniotic fluid is the liquid that cushions and protects the baby during pregnancy. When there's too much extra urine from the baby going into the amniotic fluid, it can lead to an increase in the overall volume of the amniotic fluid. This condition of having too much amniotic fluid is called "polyhydramnios." Polyhydramnios can sometimes be a sign that something is not quite right with the pregnancy, and it may require further monitoring and management by a healthcare provider. It's important for the healthcare team to keep a close eye on both the mother and the baby in such situations to ensure a healthy pregnancy and delivery. In severe cases of fetal hyperglycemia, when the baby's blood sugar levels are extremely high and not properly managed, there is an increased risk of stillbirth. Stillbirth refers to the death of the baby in the womb after 20 weeks of pregnancy but before delivery. High blood glucose levels in the baby can lead to complications that may affect the baby's health and survival.

- **Congenital Abnormalities**: Fetal hyperglycemia may increase the risk of congenital abnormalities. Congenital abnormalities are structural or functional abnormalities present in a baby at birth. Some of these congenital abnormalities include hypoglycemia, heart defects, neural tube defects, respiratory distress syndrome, and macrosomia. These abnormalities may affect various parts of the baby's body, such as the heart, spine, limbs, or other organs. The exact nature and severity of these abnormalities can vary widely.

Infant Complications of Gestational Diabetes:
Complications for the baby tend to occur during delivery or immediately after birth.

- **Macrosomia**: Since the baby is larger than normal (macrosomia), there's a higher risk of birth trauma, which can affect both the baby and the mother's genital tract.
- **Hypoglycemia**: Hypoglycemia is a medical term that refers to a condition characterized by abnormally low levels of glucose (sugar) in the bloodstream. After birth, the baby will no longer receive glucose from the mother because the umbilical cord is clamped. However, due to fetal hyperinsulinemia (increased insulin production in the fetus), the baby may experience hypoglycemia as insulin keeps shoving glucose into the cells of the baby without a new supply.
- **Hyperbilirubinemia**: Infants born to mothers with gestational diabetes have an increased risk of developing hyperbilirubinemia. Hyperbilirubinemia is a medical condition characterized by an abnormally high level of *bilirubin* in the bloodstream. Bilirubin is a yellow pigment that is produced when red blood cells are worn out and degrade. It is typically processed by the liver and then excreted from the body. When there is an excess of bilirubin in the blood, it can lead to a yellowing of the skin and the whites of the eyes, a condition known as jaundice. Here's a detailed explanation of hyperbilirubinemia:

Bilirubin Production: Bilirubin is a natural byproduct of the breakdown of old red blood cells in the body. These cells have a limited lifespan, and when they are removed from circulation, their hemoglobin (a protein in red blood cells) is broken down, leading to the formation of bilirubin.

Liver Processing: Once bilirubin is formed, it is transported to the liver, where it undergoes a series of chemical changes to make it water-soluble and easier to excrete from the body. The liver then converts this modified bilirubin into *bile*, which is a digestive fluid.

Bile Excretion: The bile containing bilirubin is stored in the gallbladder until it is needed to aid in digestion. During digestion, the bile is released into the small intestine to help break down fats. Bilirubin is eventually eliminated from the body through the stool.

Hyperbilirubinemia occurs when there is an imbalance between the formation of bilirubin and the liver's ability to process and excrete it. Infants born to mothers with gestational diabetes have an increased risk of developing hyperbilirubinemia for several reasons:

1. **Higher Birth Weight:** Babies born to mothers with gestational diabetes are more likely to be larger than average (a condition called macrosomia). Larger babies often have more red blood cells, which can break down more quickly, leading to increased bilirubin production.

2. **Polycythemia:** A condition characterized by an excess of red blood cells in the baby's bloodstream. Babies of mothers with gestational diabetes can be at an increased risk of polycythemia due to elevated blood sugar levels in the mother, which can stimulate the baby's body to produce more red blood cells.

As these extra red blood cells break down, they release more bilirubin into the baby's bloodstream.

3.**Immature Liver Function:** In some cases, infants born to mothers with gestational diabetes may have slightly immature liver function, which can slow down the processing and elimination of bilirubin. This can lead to an accumulation of bilirubin in the baby's blood.

- **Genetic Factors**: There may be genetic factors that make some infants more prone to hyperbilirubinemia, and these factors could coincide with the presence of gestational diabetes.
- **Respiratory Distress Syndrome (RDS)**: Some infants may be at an increased risk of developing respiratory distress syndrome, a condition where the baby has difficulty breathing. However, this condition is manageable.
- **Long-Term Risk**: Babies born to mothers with gestational diabetes may have an increased long-term risk of developing childhood obesity.

Risk Factors for Gestational Diabetes Mellitus (GDM) Before Pregnancy:

Now let's discuss the several factors that can increase the chances of a woman getting gestational diabetes. If a woman is exposed to these factors before pregnancy, then she has an increased risk of developing gestational diabetes during pregnancy.

1.**Overweight or Obesity**

Overweight, or obesity, is a well-established risk factor for developing gestational diabetes. When a woman is overweight or obese, it means that she has an excess amount of body fat, particularly *visceral fat,* which is located around the abdominal area and organs. This excess fat is a hallmark of insulin resistance.

In individuals who are overweight or obese, their body's fat cells, known as adipose cells, release substances called adipokines, which can be pro-inflammatory. These adipokines can disrupt the body's ability to use insulin properly, leading to a condition called insulin resistance. Additionally, the excess fat in the body can release free fatty acids into the bloodstream, further worsening the problem of insulin resistance.

Note:

- ***Visceral fat***

Visceral fat is a type of fat that is stored deep within the abdominal cavity, surrounding vital organs such as the liver, pancreas, and intestines. Unlike subcutaneous fat, which is the fat found just under the skin and can be pinched with your fingers, visceral fat is not visible from the outside. It is often referred to as "belly fat" and can pose health risks because it secretes various chemicals and hormones that can contribute to health problems, including insulin resistance, inflammation, and an increased risk of cardiovascular disease, diabetes, and other metabolic disorders. Reducing visceral fat through a healthy diet and regular physical activity is important for maintaining good health.

- ***Adipose tissue***

Adipose tissue, commonly known as fat tissue, is a specialized type of connective tissue found throughout the body whose primary function is to store excess glucose in the form of fat. It's made up of special fat cells called adipocytes. Adipose tissues are located directly beneath the skin. It is found in numerous areas of the body. Some areas where we commonly find adipose tissues are the abdomen, thighs, buttocks, hips, upper arms, and back.

When you eat more calories than your body needs, your body converts these extra calories to fats and stores them in these fat cells. This stored fat can be used for energy later, when your body needs it. Adipose tissue also helps protect and cushion your organs and keeps your body temperature steady.

- **Adipokines**

Adipokines are special proteins produced by fat cells (adipose tissue) in your body. These proteins can act like messengers and have various jobs. Some of them help control your metabolism and how your body uses energy, while others can affect inflammation or even your appetite. They play a role in how your body manages its weight and overall health. Think of them as little signals that fat cells use to communicate with the rest of your body and influence different processes.

- **Proinflammatory**

"Proinflammatory" means something that promotes or triggers inflammation in the body. Inflammation is a natural response of the immune system to protect against infections and injuries. However, when something is described as proinflammatory, it means that it encourages or intensifies this inflammatory response, which can sometimes be harmful if it becomes chronic or excessive. So, proinflammatory substances or factors can cause or worsen inflammation in the body's tissues, potentially leading to health issues.

- **Fatty acids**

Fatty acids are organic molecules that consist of a chain of carbon atoms bonded together, with hydrogen atoms attached to the carbon atoms. These molecules are a fundamental component of fats and oils. They play crucial roles in energy storage, cellular structure, and as building blocks for various biological molecules in organisms.

When a woman who is overweight or obese becomes pregnant, the hormonal changes and increased demands on her body can make the insulin resistance worse. Pregnancy hormones, especially those produced by the placenta, can amplify the insulin resistance that is already present in overweight or obese individuals. This means that more insulin is needed to keep blood sugar levels in check during pregnancy.

If the pancreas can't make enough insulin to compensate for the increased insulin resistance, blood sugar levels can rise, resulting in gestational diabetes. The combination of excess weight and insulin resistance creates a challenging situation for the body to effectively regulate blood sugar levels during pregnancy.
Furthermore, it's important to note that many overweight or obese individuals may already have underlying metabolic issues, such as impaired glucose tolerance (IGT) or prediabetes, even before they become pregnant. These pre-existing conditions make them more susceptible to developing gestational diabetes when they do become pregnant. So in summary, being overweight or obese, along with the associated insulin resistance and pre-existing metabolic problems, can increase the risk of gestational diabetes during pregnancy.

Note
- Impaired Glucose Tolerance (IGT)

Impaired Glucose Tolerance (IGT) is a condition related to how your body processes sugar (glucose) from the food you eat. In IGT, your blood sugar levels are higher than normal but not quite high enough to be considered diabetes. It's like the middle ground between normal blood sugar and diabetes.
When you have IGT, your body has a harder time using insulin (a hormone that helps control blood sugar), and your blood sugar levels can become elevated after eating.

People with IGT are at an increased risk of developing type 2 diabetes in the future, so it's a sign that you should pay attention to your diet and lifestyle to help prevent diabetes. It is important to note that the relationship between obesity and gestational diabetes is not solely based on insulin resistance. Other factors associated with obesity, such as chronic low-grade inflammation and altered adipokine secretion, can contribute to the development of gestational diabetes.

To mitigate the risks associated with overweight, obesity, and gestational diabetes, it is crucial for women to maintain a healthy weight before and during pregnancy. This includes adopting a balanced and nutritious diet, engaging in regular physical activity, and working closely with healthcare professionals to manage weight and blood sugar levels effectively. By addressing and managing weight-related factors, the incidence of gestational diabetes can be reduced, promoting better maternal and fetal health outcomes.

- **Family History**

Family history plays a significant role in the risk of developing gestational diabetes. If a woman has a close family member, such as a parent or sibling, who has been diagnosed with diabetes, particularly type 2 diabetes, her risk of developing gestational diabetes is higher.

The influence of family history on gestational diabetes risk implies a genetic predisposition to ***impaired glucose metabolism***. Specific genetic variants can contribute to insulin resistance, impaired insulin secretion, or both, making individuals more susceptible to developing diabetes, including gestational diabetes.

Genetic factors can influence various aspects of glucose metabolism. For instance, certain gene variants may impact insulin receptor function, leading to reduced sensitivity to insulin.

This results in a decreased ability of cells to take up glucose effectively, leading to elevated blood sugar levels. Other genetic variations may affect the functioning of pancreatic cells responsible for insulin production, further contributing to the risk of gestational diabetes.

It's important to note that having a family history of diabetes does not guarantee the development of gestational diabetes. Many individuals with a family history of diabetes do not develop the condition. However, a family history should alert healthcare providers to closely monitor and assess a woman's risk during pregnancy.

Knowing about a family history of diabetes allows healthcare professionals to implement preventive measures and provide targeted care. Pregnant women with a family history of diabetes may undergo earlier and more frequent screening for gestational diabetes to monitor their blood sugar levels. They may also receive counseling on healthy lifestyle modifications, such as maintaining a balanced diet, engaging in regular physical activity, and achieving a healthy weight before and during pregnancy.

Understanding the influence of family history on gestational diabetes risk helps healthcare providers identify high-risk individuals and provide appropriate management strategies. By addressing genetic and environmental factors, the aim is to minimize the risk and potential complications associated with gestational diabetes for both the mother and the baby.

Note

Impaired glucose metabolism

Impaired glucose metabolism refers to a condition in which the body has difficulty processing and regulating glucose (sugar) effectively. It is a broad term that encompasses various stages of glucose-related disorders, ranging from mild abnormalities to more severe conditions like diabetes.

In cases of impaired glucose metabolism, the body may have trouble maintaining normal blood sugar levels after consuming carbohydrates. This can manifest as higher-than-normal fasting blood sugar levels or elevated blood sugar levels after meals. While impaired glucose metabolism is not as severe as diabetes, it indicates that the body's ability to utilize insulin (a hormone that helps regulate blood sugar) is compromised.

Impaired glucose metabolism often serves as a warning sign or a precursor to more serious conditions like prediabetes or type 2 diabetes. It highlights the need for lifestyle modifications, including dietary changes and increased physical activity, to prevent the progression of diabetes and maintain optimal blood sugar control.

Risk factors for developing GDM during pregnancy.
The risk factors listed below can increase a woman's risk of getting gestational diabetes during her pregnant phase.

1. **Maternal Age**: Pregnant women aged 35 years or older have an increased risk of GDM.
2. **Polycystic Ovarian Syndrome (PCOS)**: Polycystic Ovarian Syndrome (PCOS) is a hormonal disorder that affects women, often leading to irregular menstrual cycles, excessive production of androgens (male hormones), and the formation of small fluid-filled sacs (cysts) in the ovaries. Several studies show that PCOS increases the risk of insulin resistance and can potentially lead to gestational diabetes.
3. **Ethnicity**: Certain ethnic groups, including Southeast Asians, have a higher predisposition to GDM.
4. **Previous GDM**: If a woman has had a previous pregnancy with GDM, there is a greater likelihood of experiencing it in subsequent pregnancies.

Why is Diabetes a Concern?
Globally, diabetes is a major public health hazard that has reached alarming levels that are comparable to an epidemic. Chronic, noncommunicable diseases like diabetes and hypertension are becoming more common, and they account for approximately 18 million deaths from cardiovascular disease each year.

The increasing number of overweight and obese people worldwide approaching 1.7 billion adults and 155 million children is closely linked to this rise. According to estimates from the International Diabetes Federation, the number of people with diabetes will increase from 246 million to 380 million by 2025, with the prevalence of the disease estimated to reach 7.3% from 8.0% in 2007. In a similar vein, rates of impaired glucose tolerance (IGT) were 7.5% in 2007 and are predicted to drop to 6.0% by 2025, impacting an additional 418 million people worldwide from 308 million in 2007.

The burden is borne by developing countries, where more than 80% of adults with diabetes live. With 9.2% of the adult population affected, the Eastern Mediterranean and Middle East have the highest incidence rates, followed by North America with 8.4%. The Western Pacific region leads in absolute numbers, with 67 million people diagnosed with diabetes, followed by Europe with 53 million, despite lower prevalence rates. Interestingly, with 40.9 million and 39.8 million people with diabetes, respectively, India and China lead the world's top ten lists. The United States, Russia, Germany, Japan, Pakistan, Brazil, Mexico, and Egypt are the next most populous countries on the list.
Two major issues with the rising prevalence of diabetes are that

most of the rise is expected to come from developing countries and that type 2 diabetes is emerging at an alarmingly early age, especially in fat children who are not yet in puberty. Diabetes usually affects people beyond retirement age in developed countries, but in developing nations, the majority of individuals affected are between the ages of 35 and 64 and are in the midst of their productive lives.

In Asian countries, the risk of type 2 diabetes tends to rise sharply at BMI levels considered manageable for white people in Europe and North America. A suggestion has been made to create specific obesity classifications for Asians, with BMI 23 being considered overweight and BMI 25 or 27 being obese. The estimated 250 million individuals who are obese globally, according to current estimates, might be significantly impacted by implementing these changes.

Seven million people worldwide are diagnosed with diabetes each year, with type 2 diabetes rates rising most sharply in areas where rapid and significant lifestyle changes are occurring. This demonstrates the vital significance of lifestyle factors and emphasizes the potential to reverse the global diabetes epidemic. People who have type 2 diabetes are two to four times more likely to develop cardiovascular disease, and an astounding eighty percent of diabetics will eventually pass away from cardiovascular issues. An estimated 12 to 14 years of life are lost due to diabetes-related early mortality. In addition, the costs associated with treating diabetic patients are two to five times higher than those without the condition.

According to estimates from the World Health Organization, diabetes-related diseases account for as much as 15% of annual health expenditures. According to global estimates, the annual direct healthcare costs associated with diabetes among people aged 20 to 79 amounts to as much as $286 billion.

The growing incidence of type 2 diabetes has significant negative effects on the economy and society, which emphasizes the urgent need for prevention measures.

The best way to avoid the effects of type 2 diabetes may be to take preventative measures before the disease even starts. Diabetes is very expensive for those who have it and their families, as well as for healthcare systems, because of its chronic nature and the severity of its effects. Increased blood sugar levels are the hallmark of many common metabolic diseases, collectively referred to as diabetes mellitus (DM). Different types of diabetes mellitus (DM) arise due to the intricate interplay between genetic, environmental, and lifestyle factors.

Within a generation or two, economic progress in low- and middle-income countries often alters living conditions, including diet and physical activity levels. As a result, people may develop diabetes even with very modest weight increases. On the other hand, diabetes affects the poorest populations more often in developed countries. However, in both settings, poverty and poor sanitation contribute to a higher prevalence of type 2 diabetes by pushing families toward inexpensive, high-calorie meals and packaged beverages.

The identification of some genes that predispose people to type 2 diabetes has advanced significantly. The identification of susceptibility genes provides new targets for drug development in addition to enabling the early deployment of preventive measures targeted at those most at risk. Obesity ranks among the main risk factors for type 2 diabetes. Gaining weight causes insulin resistance in a number of ways. Clinical studies have shown that in the majority of obese individuals with impaired glucose tolerance, a mere 5% weight loss is sufficient to prevent the development of type 2 diabetes.

In the majority of industrialized countries, diabetes is the fourth-leading cause of death. Diabetes-related complications include peripheral vascular disease, heart attacks, diabetic neuropathy, amputations, kidney failure, and blindness. These conditions also lead to an increase in disability, a reduction in life expectancy, and significant healthcare costs for almost every society. Diabetes will thus always rank among the most important health issues of the twenty-first century.

An estimated 3.2 million individuals worldwide lose their lives to diabetes every year. Diabetes patients suffer greatly from heart disease, often without realizing it. Fifty to eighty percent of deaths connected to diabetes are caused by cardiovascular disease. One of the most frequent side effects is diabetic neuropathy, and the main cause of blindness and visual impairment is diabetes retinopathy.

Studies show that after 15 years of diabetes, around 2% of people have blindness, and about 10% have significant visual impairment. One of the main causes of renal failure is diabetes, whose incidence varies by demography and is correlated with the severity and prognosis of the illness. Diabetes is the most prevalent cause of non-traumatic lower-limb amputations.

Diabetic foot sickness is caused by vascular and nerve abnormalities, which often culminate in ulceration and later limb amputation. The "metabolic syndrome," which comprises obesity, insulin resistance, and other cardiovascular risk factors, is often linked to type 2 diabetes. The significance of early and aggressive treatment for insulin resistance, dyslipidemia, hypertension, and albuminuria is highlighted by recent advancements in type 2 diabetes medication. The use of second-generation oral medications, home glucose and glycohemoglobin monitoring, recombinant human insulin, and a deeper understanding of the connection between complications and diabetic management have all been developments in the previous ten years in the treatment of diabetes. In addition, it has been rediscovered how effective continuous subcutaneous insulin infusion, or pump therapy, is.

In the near future, the creation of new insulins has the potential to significantly enhance insulin treatment regimens by enabling more accurate modeling of endogenous insulin function. Oral and inhaled formulations are particularly important because they provide patient-friendly alternatives that may help a larger population of diabetics achieve better glucose control. Clinical studies have shown that for both type 1 and type 2 diabetes, inhaled insulin is just as effective as injectable normal insulin.
Additionally, an oral insulin spray that is quickly absorbed via the buccal mucosa is being studied in current clinical studies as a potential additional non-injected insulin option.

Numerous novel insulin analogs are anticipated to aid in the management of both type 1 and type 2 diabetes. Glitazones target the nuclear hormone receptor PPARy, or peroxisome proliferator-activated receptor, which controls lipid and glucose metabolism. Currently, medications that target this receptor as well as another receptor that is related to fat metabolism and that fibrates also target are being explored. In the next few years, it is anticipated that these dual PPARy/a agonists will play a significant role in managing type 2 diabetes and metabolic syndrome. Clinical investigations have shown that the lipase inhibitor orlistat, which is mostly used to treat obesity, has positive results as an insulin-sensitizing medication that also aids in weight management. Gut-derived hormones known as incretins, such as gastric inhibitory peptide and glucagon-like peptide-1 (GLP-1),   50 are examples of insulin secretagogues. Clinical trials are now testing GLP-1 analogues and receptor agonists, which may prove to be highly helpful for diabetes patients.

A major advancement has been made with the recent implementation of continuous blood glucose monitoring devices. Through non-invasive technologies like reverse iontophoresis, which draws glucose molecules through the skin and collects them in a gel disc using a low electric current, these devices give frequent automated glucose readings. Financial constraints have prevented the widespread usage of a wristwatch-like gadget that has been approved for patients over seven in the United States.
For evaluating the effectiveness of diabetes treatment, the glycosylated hemoglobin (HbA1c) test remains the gold standard.

With the demands of vigorous treatment on patients and their families, particularly in adolescence, it is essential to expedite assessment and education via the use of desktop devices for rapid measurement. Pediatric diabetes care has greatly benefited from advances in insulin therapy, including the use of programmable pumps for automated administration of insulin and the development of novel insulins. Soon, a fully automated "closed-loop" system with algorithmic insulin delivery via a pump and real-time glucose testing will be available.

Furthermore, type 1 diabetes treatment options include islet and stem cell transplantation, as well as studies into controlling the autoimmune reaction. Treatment-wise, islet cell transplantation seems promising. This minimally invasive procedure includes perfusing isolated islet cells from cadaver pancreases into the portal vein.

Finding the elusive type 1 diabetes trigger or triggers may pave the way for prophylactic measures that might reduce the disease's incidence worldwide. New insulin analogs that allow more physiological insulin delivery have been made possible by developments in recombinant DNA technology. Future insulin treatment processes may see the use of inhaled and oral insulin formulations in place of several injections. Currently, a number of research labs are investigating noninvasive glucose monitoring technologies, such as infrared radiation spectroscopy. Many companies are investigating devices that use less intrusive techniques, such as transdermal patches and microneedles, to measure interstitial fluid glucose, much like the Glucowatch.

Although clinical settings are being used to evaluate interstitial fluid extraction devices, most noninvasive infrared technologies still need to be improved. Although long-term, stable implanted glucose sensor research is still in its infancy, it is thought to be essential for the development of future artificial pancreases. The growing prevalence of diabetes demands immediate attention, and prevention seems to be a viable approach. It has been shown that making lifestyle modifications, including losing weight and engaging in moderate exercise, may reduce the occurrence of diabetes in those with impaired glucose tolerance by more than half. Metformin, acarbose, and other drugs are useful in preventing type 2 diabetes in high-risk individuals with insulin-glucose intolerance, according to randomized prospective trials. Preventing issues may be best achieved through intervention prior to the onset of type 2 diabetes. Unquestionably, clinical research has shown that lowering LDL cholesterol and blood pressure in diabetics may help prevent heart disease and stroke.

Not only is diabetes preventable, but it also works. Research suggests that decreasing 5 to 7 percent of body weight may help people who are at high risk of type 2 diabetes prevent or delay the onset of the condition. The widespread use of fasting plasma glucose (FPG) as a type 2 diabetes screening test is advised by the American Diabetes Association (ADA). Every three years, the ADA advises screening all adults over 45, with early screening recommended for individuals with extra-risk factors. By using prompt and consistent monitoring strategies, problems associated with diabetes may be significantly decreased. All diabetics should get these tests. In addition, annual screening for hypertension and dyslipidemia is advised. People with diabetes should have annual influenza vaccinations as well as pneumococcal and tetanus vaccinations at recommended intervals, in addition to basic medical treatment. A lot of diabetics may think about using aspirin. Governments must have a strong political will to create policies that support lifestyle modifications in order to prevent type 2 diabetes. The United Nations General Assembly recognized diabetes as a chronic, costly, and crippling condition that has major ramifications for families, governments, and the world at large when it voted on a historic resolution on December 20, 2006.

The real winners from this agreement will be those who have diabetes, their families, and those who are vulnerable. All countries must ratify the UN Resolution and implement national diabetes prevention programs that serve the whole populace. Both self-screening and opportunistic screening by medical experts may be useful in identifying those who are at a high risk of developing type 2 diabetes.

Numerous studies carried out in various nations have shown substantial evidence about the effectiveness of lifestyle modifications, such as maintaining a healthy body weight and engaging in moderate physical activity, in preventing type 2 diabetes among those at high risk.

Education on a balanced diet and the need for exercise is crucial for managing diabetes and maintaining a healthy lifestyle. Action must be taken right now due to the increasing strain diabetes is placing on healthcare systems and the global economy. Individualized care plans are necessary, and they must cover concerns including managing weight, stopping smoking, and maintaining psychological well-being, in addition to taking into consideration cultural, age-related, and self-care skills. Sustaining the predicted global increase in diabetes prevalence—especially in developing countries—requires enough resources, in addition to treating early-onset insulin-dependent diabetic mellitus and preventing the complications of diabetes later in life.

Numerous pharmacological medicines are now being evaluated in large prospective studies, suggesting that one or more of these approaches may soon make diabetes prevention a reality.
Advances in our understanding of the molecular mechanisms connecting obesity to insulin resistance will direct the development of novel therapeutic targets for the prevention and treatment of type 2 diabetes.

Researchers are working hard to identify all the genetic and environmental factors, such as viruses, toxins, and dietary effects, that contribute to type 1 diabetes in order to prevent or treat the autoimmune death of insulin-producing cells.
Researchers will be able to assess the effectiveness of presently being explored medicines and preventive measures, as well as get a better understanding of the sickness process with the use of imaging tools for beta cells that safely create insulin. Emerging technology, such as closed-loop devices that automatically measure blood glucose levels and adjust insulin dosage, will soon be available. With so much data at our disposal, specialized treatments may be created to prevent diabetic related issues.

A component of life is responsibility; life is a journey full of constant change and challenges. Taking little steps to delay or prevent the onset of the illness and live a long, healthy life will pay off big time.

TYPE 2 Diabetes

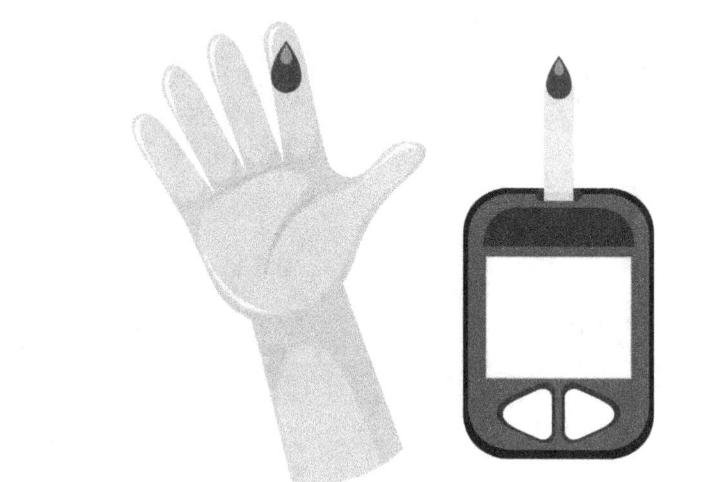

N. KEHSENI
MARKBRON

CHAPTER ONE

What Is Type 2 Diabetes?

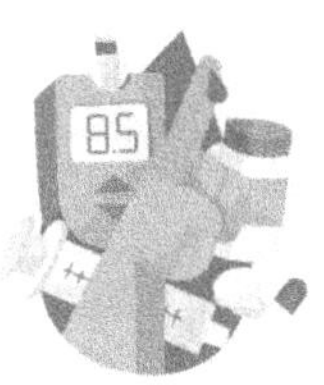

If you have been paying close attention, at this stage you should be able to understand the nature of type 1 and gestational diabetes and how they work. However, in this particular chapter, we aim to discuss type 2 diabetes, which is highly prevalent and constitutes about 90-95% of diabetic cases. That is precisely why we have dedicated a separate chapter to it. Now, let's examine the definition of type 2 diabetes and understand how it comes about.

Type 2 diabetes is a chronic metabolic disease characterized by high blood sugar levels due to a condition known as **insulin resistance.** Insulin resistance is a condition whereby the cells of the body exhibit reduced responsiveness to the effects of insulin, a hormone produced by the pancreas.

When the cells of the body exhibit reduced responsiveness to insulin, they are not able to open up effectively for the absorption of glucose. Remember that insulin acts as a key that opens up the cell for glucose to go in and be used for energy production.

Unlike type 1 diabetes, whose underlying mechanism is autoimmune destruction of the pancreatic beta cells, the underlying mechanism behind type 2 diabetes is insulin resistance. Which we intend to break down for you in the most simple and effective way.

In order to have a flawless understanding of type 2 diabetes and grasp the concept behind insulin resistance, let's have a little recap on how the food that you eat is being converted into energy by cells to use for your daily activities and how type 2 diabetes impairs this function. 57

Glucose Metabolism

After consuming food that contains carbohydrates, the enzymes in your small intestine break down these carbohydrates into single sugar molecules, such as glucose. The lining of your small intestine absorbs the glucose and transfers it into the bloodstream. When the blood reaches your pancreas, specialized cells within the pancreas known as beta cells detect the rise in blood sugar levels and release insulin into the bloodstream.

Another hormone called ***glucagon-like peptide-1 (GLP-1)*** helps the pancreas produce the right amount of insulin. GLP-1 is released from the intestines in response to the presence of food, particularly carbohydrates, which maintain glucose homeostasis in the body.

Note:

Glucagon-like peptide-1 (GLP-1) is a hormone released from the intestines in response to the presence of food, particularly carbohydrates. GLP-1 plays a crucial role in regulating blood sugar levels by helping the pancreas produce the right amount of insulin. Here's how it functions:

1. Food Intake: When you eat, especially when you consume carbohydrates, the digestive process begins in the stomach and continues into the small intestine.
2. Release of GLP-1: GLP-1-secreting cells in the intestines detect the presence of nutrients, particularly glucose and fatty acids, as a result of digestion. In response to these nutrients, these cells release GLP-1 into the bloodstream.
3. Blood Sugar Regulation: GLP-1 has several important functions. Some of which include;

- ***Insulin Release****: It stimulates the pancreas to release insulin. Insulin helps regulate blood sugar levels by facilitating the uptake of glucose by cells, reducing blood sugar levels.*
- ***Slows Gastric Emptying****: GLP-1 also slows down the emptying of the stomach, which can help control the rate at which nutrients, including glucose, are absorbed into the bloodstream.*
- ***Satiety****: GLP-1 has been associated with feelings of fullness and satiety after eating, which can contribute to reduced food intake and weight management.*

Insulin-Mediated Glucose Uptake.

As blood circulates throughout your body, the secreted insulin, together with glucose, exits the bloodstream and enters your body's tissues to reach the cells. Each cell utilizes glucose as its primary source of energy for various metabolic processes.

The process of glucose entering a cell can be compared to a lock-and-key mechanism. Every cell in your body possesses insulin receptors on its surface, which act as locks. Insulin acts as the key that unlocks the cell, allowing glucose to enter. Once inside the cell, the glucose undergoes a series of processes to produce energy, enabling the cell to function properly.

Individuals with type 2 diabetes experience a condition known as insulin resistance, which compromises the mechanism of glucose intake by the body cells, resulting in high blood sugar levels. In this condition, the cells of the body are resisting the effects of insulin, and as such, they refuse to open up for glucose to get into the cells, causing glucose to stockpile in the bloodstream, a condition known as hyperglycemia. Hyperglycemia (high blood glucose) is a major criterion for diagnosing diabetes.

What Is Insulin Resistance?

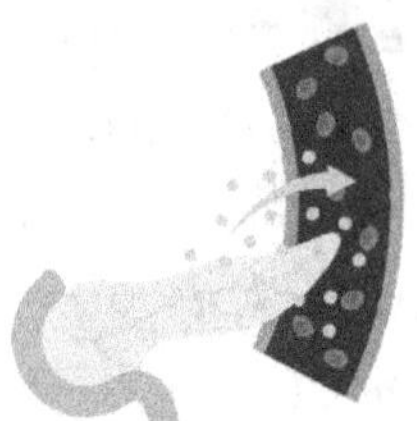

Insulin resistance is the underlying mechanism of prediabetes and type 2 diabetes. also, the most important process to grasp in order to have a very good understanding of how type 2 diabetes comes about. It is so important to discuss insulin resistance because it is linked to the **metabolic syndrome.**

Note:

The metabolic syndrome is a cluster of conditions that occur together, increasing the risk of heart disease, stroke, and type 2 diabetes. The presence of metabolic syndrome is typically diagnosed when an individual has a combination of several key factors related to cardiovascular health and metabolism. The specific criteria for diagnosing metabolic syndrome may vary slightly between different health organizations, but they generally include a combination of the following:

- *Central Obesity*
- *Elevated blood pressure*
- *High Blood Sugar (Insulin Resistance)*
- *High Triglyceride Levels*
- *Low HDL cholesterol levels*

Over the years, a lot of studies have been conducted in an attempt to explain insulin resistance. Insulin resistance has been a topic of discussion in the medical field for years now, and this is because many explanations trying to elucidate this condition somehow don't add up. But in this section, we are going to look at two of the most controversial and discussed theories behind insulin resistance. We are equally going to look at a detailed yet simple explanation of insulin resistance and how it has helped to improve our knowledge of diabetes over the years.

Now, when a person is diagnosed with type 2 diabetes, high levels of glucose are found in their bloodstream, which is the primary criterion for diagnosing diabetes. We could be tempted to think that there is an absence of insulin as in type 1 diabetes, but when the insulin levels are measured, they are found to be present and in very large amounts in the early stages of type 2 diabetes. This is because the pancreas is relentlessly producing higher levels of insulin in an attempt to compensate for the insulin resistance exhibited by the cells of the body. This tells us that the problem doesn't come from a lack of insulin but from the way the cells in our body utilize the insulin being produced. Then we ask ourselves, Why are the cells resisting the effects of insulin? Why is glucose not getting into the cells as it should?

1. Lock and key mechanism

For many years, we have looked at insulin resistance as a problem with the insulin receptors found on the cells and insulin itself, stating that the reason why the body cell doesn't absorb glucose is because the insulin receptors (lock) on the cells are gummed up, therefore implying that insulin (key) is unable to unlock the cells for the intake of glucose. Some theories even propose that the insulin receptors have changed shape and are no longer compatible with insulin, causing glucose to stockpile in the blood stream. Now we ask ourselves. "What's gumming up the cell? What could have possibly caused the insulin receptors to change shape?

Several studies propose that as an individual gains a lot of weight, the fats present in their body will start building up in their internal organs, notably around the liver. However, as this happens, these fats will infiltrate the cells of these organs and block the insulin signaling pathways (receptors) through a series of processes that prevent glucose metabolism.

Such that when insulin binds to the insulin receptors, the cells do not open up, preventing glucose from going in and leading to the accumulation of glucose in the blood streams. This explanation is very convincing at first glance, but it is not entirely true for the following reasons:

Discrepancy Between Expected and Observed Weight changes

If we go by the hypothesis stated above, it will imply that there will be very high levels of glucose in the blood stream and little or no glucose in the cells. Due to low levels of glucose in the cells, they should start experiencing a condition known as *internal starvation*, causing the patient to lose a lot of weight due to processes like Lipolysis(the breakdown of fats for energy), but this is unlike what we see in Type 2 diabetes patients. Type 2 diabetes patients tend to experience a lot of weight gain and develop abdominal obesity instead of losing weight.

Note:

Internal Starvation:

Internal starvation is a term used to describe a condition that occurs when there is a deficiency of glucose inside the cells of the body. This condition arises when glucose, which is a primary source of energy for cells, cannot effectively enter the cells, often due to factors like insulin resistance or insufficient insulin production,

- ## Insulin receptor imaging

When we examine the structure of the insulin receptors found on the cells of the body in a type 2 diabetic patient using insulin receptor imaging, we see that they have not changed shape, nor are they gummed up, but rather are few in number. This implies that they are indeed working, but for some reason they're showing reduced responsiveness to the effects of insulin, not that they are gummed up or have changed shape.

- **Polyphagia (increased hunger):**

Another reason why the lock and key mechanism is faulty in trying to explain insulin resistance is that if we go by that mechanism, it makes sense that since there is little to no glucose in the cells due to the fact that the insulin receptors are faulty, as this mechanism proposes, we would normally expect that the low glucose would lead to low energy being produced, as the cell is responsible for producing energy.

This low energy should, in turn, lead to an excessive amount of hunger, as we see in type 1 diabetes. If glucose is truly not present in the cell, then the starving cells will push the brain to secrete hunger hormones to encourage you to eat more and more, as we see in type 1 diabetes.

But what we notice in type 2 diabetes is that only a very small percentage of type 2 diabetes patients actually experience frequent hunger, and we will see why this happens as we continue with our study on diabetes.

- **Diabetic ketoacidosis (DKA)**

Another reason why this lock and key mechanism fails in an attempt to explain insulin resistance is a condition known as diabetic ketoacidosis (DKA). Diabetic ketoacidosis (DKA) is a serious and potentially life-threatening complication that can occur in people with diabetes, usually type 1 diabetes. It develops when the body doesn't have enough insulin to properly use glucose for energy, so it starts breaking down fat for energy instead. This process releases ketones, which builds up in the blood. Ketones are chemical substances produced by the liver during the breakdown of fat for energy. They are an alternative source of fuel when there is not enough glucose (sugar) available for energy. It is important to note that dangerously high levels of ketones in the blood are very dangerous and can have severe consequences.

- Now, if we try to go by the lock and key mechanism in an attempt to explain what insulin resistance is, we see that diabetic ketoacidosis should be a very active and common complication of type 2 diabetes. This is because, given that the insulin receptors are not working and glucose can't get into the cells, we should normally have the body break down fat cells for energy. This would not only cause weight loss and polyphagia, as we have seen in type 1 diabetes, but also cause the release of these ketone bodies in the blood.

- But what do we see with type 2 diabetes? When testing for the presence of ketones in the blood of type 2 diabetes patients, we notice that there is an absence of ketone bodies in their blood. This simply tells us that the insulin receptors are not completely jammed or dysfunctional as this mechanism proposes, because if that were the case, the body would effectively turn to fats for energy, and we know that the byproduct of the breakdown of fats for energy produces ketone bodies, and as we have seen, these ketone bodies are absent in type 2 diabetes patients. So somehow, the insulin receptors are working, but glucose is stockpiling in the bloodstream and hardly getting into the cells. And this explanation tells us clearly that the lock-and-key paradigm of insulin resistance is wrong.

Note

Diabetic ketoacidosis is actually very, very rare among type 2 diabetes individuals and is not as common as it is in type 1 diabetes, where the cells are actually starving and the body has to turn to alternative energy sources like fats.

Now, after realizing that this lock and key mechanism of insulin resistance is faulty, the big question still remains. WHAT THEN CAUSES INSULIN RESISTANCE?

2. Overflow mechanism

Every biological system always tries to be in a homeostatic state, that is, a state of balance or equilibrium among all biological systems required for them to survive and function properly. The human body is also a biological system, and it constantly tries to be in a homeostatic state.

This therefore means that if you have excessive amounts of any substance in your body, say glucose, the body will try to regulate the excess. There are several ways in which the body can regulate the excess of any substance. but one of the most common ways will be to store the excess amount of this substance. The body does all this in an attempt to return to a balanced and homeostatic state. Now, when the body starts receiving an exaggerated amount of this substance, say glucose, the body will start showing signs of resistance toward that substance as it already has enough of this particular substance in its system. This resistance also occurs because the body is desperately trying to return to a homeostatic state.

Now, using this explanation, let's define what causes insulin resistance.

Many studies have pointed out a simple and logical explanation that answers the question, "What is insulin resistance?" describing insulin resistance as an overflow of glucose, suggesting that the more you keep consuming foods rich in carbohydrate with limited physical activity to burn up glucose for a long enough period of time, the body's response to this high glucose intake will be to store up the glucose in the various storage sites (muscle, liver, adipose tissues, etc.). The insulin in your body will continuously keep pushing more and more glucose into the cells of these target organs responsible for glucose storage, day after day, year after year. These cells eventually get overfilled and get to a point where your body will have a hard time pushing any more glucose into the cells, and it would require a lot more insulin to push up more glucose in these cells. As the cells get filled and can't take up any more glucose, the body starts to develop resistance to the factor responsible for shoving up glucose in the cell, which is insulin in this case.

Now let's look at it this way, so as to facilitate understanding of this concept. When you put dirt in a dustbin, what happens is that, over time, the dustbin eventually gets full. If the dustbin is full and you want to put in more dirt without emptying it, you will have to push down the already present dirt to create more space in the dustbin for more and more dirt to be able to fit in. As the dustbin gets full, a greater push force will be needed to push down the extra dirt into the dustbin. And as you keep pushing down the dirt, you will notice that the dustbin will start resisting the push force, leading to an overflow of dirt.

To make it easier to understand, let's relate this analogy to the cells.

- **Dustbin as a Cell:** Think of your cell as a dustbin that can take in sugar (glucose).
- **Insulin as the Push Force:** Insulin acts like the force you use to push down the dirt into the dustbin.
- **Glucose as the Dirt:** Glucose is the dirt you are trying to put into the dustbin (cell).

In a healthy person, the dustbin is empty enough that there is very little to no push force needed (normal insulin levels) to fit the dirt (glucose) in the dustbin (cell).

In type 2 diabetes:

- **Full Dustbin:** Over time, the dustbin (cell) gets fuller and fuller, meaning there's already a lot of glucose inside the cells, resulting from unhealthy eating habits and a lack of physical activity.
- **Need for More Force**: To put in more dirt (glucose), you need to push harder (produce more insulin).
- **Resistance:** The more you push, the more the dustbin (cell) resists. It becomes harder and harder to fit more dirt (glucose) inside. This is like the cell becoming resistant to insulin.
- **Overflow:** Eventually, the dirt (glucose) starts to overflow because the dustbin (cell) can't take in any more, no matter how hard you push (how much insulin is produced). This is like the high blood sugar levels seen in diabetes.

So, just as a full dustbin resists more dirt being added, cells in a person with type 2 diabetes resist taking in more glucose, even when there is plenty of insulin trying to help.

The same thing happens with the human body. Consuming a lot of meals rich in glucose and not doing enough physical activities to burn down the glucose will result in the glucose being stored. Now, when glucose has been stored over the years, the storage sites eventually get filled with glucose, and as such, they can no longer take up glucose for storage. And since the body wants to be in a homeostatic state, it starts resisting the effects of insulin to store up more glucose. This will result in the production of a higher-than-normal level of insulin by the pancreas to shove up more glucose into the cells of the body.

Note

The human body was not designed such that glucose should

remain in the blood stream but in the cells of the body or to be stored as fats and glycogen; therefore, as the cells of the body are resisting the effects of insulin, more and more insulin will be needed to overcome the resistance. We must keep in mind that when there is a lot of glucose in the bloodstream, it has a series of complications over time.

Reasons Why the Overflow Mechanism Works in Explaining insulin Resistance

1. Overweight

If we go by this concept, we would expect that people with this condition should be overweight (due to a high level of glucose in the cell, some of which had been converted to fats), and this is exactly what we see in most type 2 diabetic patients. They generally tend to be obese due to the accumulation of glucose over the years and little or no physical activity to burn up the glucose.

2. Fatty liver:

One of the reasons why the overflow mechanism works so well in explaining insulin resistance is because of a condition we see in type 2 diabetes patients known as fatty liver. Now, when the pancreas detects a rise in the level of glucose in the blood, the kneejerk reaction is for it to secrete insulin. After insulin shoves all of the possible glucose into the cell, it goes to the liver and tells it to convert the excess glucose to glycogen.

Note

Glycogen is like a storage form of glucose in our bodies. It's made up of lots of glucose molecules linked together in a special way suitable for storage. You can think of glycogen as multiple glucose molecules linked together, creating a compact and easily stored energy source. Whenever our body is in need of energy, it goes to the glycogen stores and converts it back.

into glucose so that they can be used up for energy. It is important to note that glycogen is mainly stored in the liver and the skeletal muscles of the body.

When glucose has been converted to glycogen and the glycogen stores are full, insulin now tells the liver to convert the excess glucose into fats. The liver, through a complex series of metabolic processes, converts this glucose into fats in a process known as **de novo lipogenesis (DNL).** These fats produced from glucose in the liver are packaged into a form suitable for transportation called **Very Low-Density Lipoproteins (VLDL)** and carried to the adipose tissues for storage. Over time, as you consume more and more glucose-rich meals, more insulin is secreted into the blood, and it goes on to tell the liver to convert all this excess glucose into fat. It gets to a point where a lot of fats are being produced by the liver, so much so that some of these fats are not transported to the adipose tissues for storage but start building up in and around the liver and accumulate over time to develop this condition known as fatty liver. It is important to note that these fats don't only build around the liver but also around internal organs such as the heart, pancreas, and kidney, which are all not suitable for fat storage and can have long-term health complications if not taken care of.

Now, if we look at insulin resistance the way the lock-and-key mechanism explains it, stating that the reason the cells of the body are resisting the effects of insulin is due to the fact that the insulin receptors have been jammed or gummed up, causing glucose to sit in the blood streams, this should imply that since the cells are resistant to insulin, little or no glucose is getting into the liver cells, and as such, there should be no production of new fat cells, and a fatty liver should not be a thing, but this is unlike what we see in type 2 diabetes.

But if we look at insulin resistance the way the overflow mechanism explains it, which is that the reason the cells of the body are resisting the effects of insulin is due to the fact that they have excess accumulated glucose through years of unhealthy eating and sedentary lifestyles, such that they have no storage space for any more glucose and are forced to resist the effects of insulin for them to take any more glucose. It makes complete sense that the liver should focus on converting all the excess glucose found within its cells and in the blood stream into fats, resulting in a fatty liver, and this is exactly what we see in type 2 diabetes. So essentially, what we see is that the high levels of insulin produced by the pancreas in response to the high levels of glucose tell the liver to convert this glucose into fats, and the liver converts so much glucose into fats that some of this fat gets stored in the liver, which shouldn't be the case as it causes this condition known as fatty liver.

What is Prediabetes?

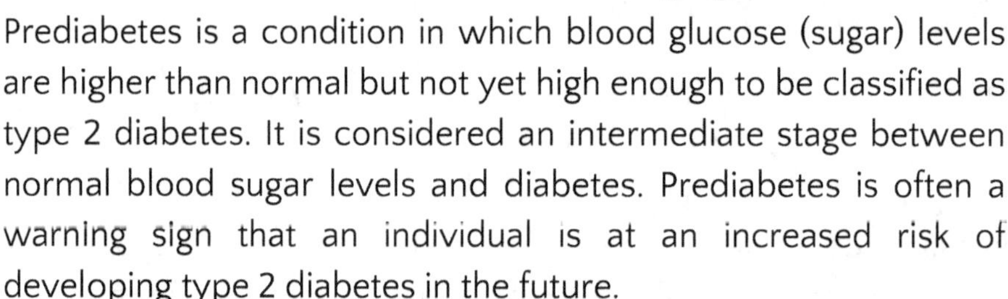

Prediabetes is a condition in which blood glucose (sugar) levels are higher than normal but not yet high enough to be classified as type 2 diabetes. It is considered an intermediate stage between normal blood sugar levels and diabetes. Prediabetes is often a warning sign that an individual is at an increased risk of developing type 2 diabetes in the future.

Just like in type 2 diabetes, the cells in your body exhibit reduced responsiveness to the actions of insulin, and this is so because an exaggerated amount of glucose has been taken up by the cells of the body again and again, and as such, the cells are packed with glucose and cannot take any more of it. And as we would expect, the pancreas will compensate for the reduced responsiveness of insulin by producing more insulin.

Over time, however, the pancreas may struggle to sustain this heightened insulin demand, causing blood sugar levels to rise over time. This elevated blood sugar level is an indication that the body's ability to regulate glucose is compromised.

With continued insulin resistance and the pancreas unable to meet the demand for insulin, blood sugar levels continue to rise. Eventually, the pancreas becomes unable to maintain normal blood sugar levels, and then you eventually develop type 2 diabetes over time.

Currently, around 88 million Americans, which is more than one-third of the population, have prediabetes. Surprisingly, about 85% of these people are not aware that they have it. Unfortunately, there are usually no clear signs or symptoms of prediabetes until it progresses and leads to future health problems.

Despite the fact that prediabetes indicates an increased risk of developing type 2 diabetes, it is also an opportunity for intervention. With appropriate lifestyle changes and, in some cases, medication, individuals with prediabetes can prevent, reverse, or delay the onset of type 2 diabetes and reduce the risk of associated complications.

There are two states in which prediabetes can manifest: impaired glucose tolerance (IGT) and impaired fasting glucose (IFG).

Impaired Glucose Tolerance (IGT)
Impaired Glucose Tolerance (IGT) is a condition characterized by elevated blood sugar levels that are higher than normal but not high enough to be diagnosed as diabetes. It typically occurs after

consuming food, especially foods high in carbohydrates.

In individuals with normal glucose tolerance, blood sugar levels rise after eating but return to normal levels relatively quickly due to the action of insulin. However, in individuals with IGT, blood sugar levels rise higher than normal after meals and may take longer to return to normal levels. This indicates that the body is having difficulty processing glucose efficiently.

Impaired Fasting Glucose (IFG)

Impaired fasting glucose (IFG) is a condition characterized by elevated blood sugar levels while fasting, indicating a reduced ability of the body to maintain normal glucose levels during periods of fasting.

When you haven't eaten for several hours, your body relies on stored glucose (glycogen) to maintain blood sugar levels. Normally, fasting blood sugar (the level of glucose in the bloodstream after an overnight fast, typically for at least 8 hours without eating.) should fall within a certain range. However, in individuals with IFG, blood sugar levels are higher than normal while fasting. And this tells us that the body has a hard time regulating blood sugar levels.

Both IGT and IFG serve as warning signs that the body's ability to regulate blood sugar is compromised. Leading to a high risk of developing type 2 diabetes over time.

Diagnosis of prediabetes

The two primary indicators used to diagnose prediabetes are *fasting plasma glucose (FPG) levels* and *hemoglobin A1c (HbA1c) levels*. Below are the diagnostic standards for prediabetes:

1. **Fasting Plasma Glucose (FPG):**

Fasting plasma glucose (FPG) is a medical test that measures the concentration of glucose (sugar) in your blood after you have fasted for a specific period, typically overnight or for at least 8 hours. It is an essential component of blood glucose monitoring and is commonly used to diagnose and manage diabetes mellitus.

Here's a detailed explanation of fasting plasma glucose (FPG):

Purpose of the Fasting Plasma Glucose (FPG) Test:

- **Diagnosis of Diabetes:** FPG is primarily used to diagnose diabetes or prediabetes. It helps determine if your blood glucose levels are within the normal range or if they are elevated, which can be an early sign of diabetes.
- **Monitoring Diabetes Management:** For individuals already diagnosed with diabetes, FPG is used to monitor how well blood sugar levels are being controlled, especially during fasting periods.

Test Procedure:

- The FPG test requires you to fast for at least 8 hours before the blood sample is taken. Typically, this means no food or drink (other than water) during the fasting period.
- A healthcare provider or a phlebotomist will draw a blood sample from a vein, usually from your arm.
- After that, the drawn blood is delivered to a lab for testing.

Normal FPG Levels:

- Normal fasting plasma glucose levels typically fall in the range of 70 to 99 milligrams per deciliter (mg/dL) of blood.

Interpretation of FPG Results:

- **Normal:** If your FPG level falls within the normal range, it indicates that your body is effectively regulating blood glucose levels, and you are not likely to have diabetes.
- **Prediabetes:** FPG levels between 100 and 125 mg/dL are indicative of prediabetes. This means you are at increased risk of developing diabetes in the future, but it is not yet diabetes.
- **Diabetes:** A diagnosis of diabetes is typically made if your FPG level is consistently 126 mg/dL or higher on two separate

occasions.

Factors Affecting FPG Levels:

- Several factors can affect FPG levels, including stress, illness, certain medications, and physical activity. Therefore, it is important to discuss these factors with your healthcare provider to interpret FPG results accurately.

Implications:

- Elevated FPG levels can indicate that your body is not properly processing glucose, which can lead to various health complications if left unmanaged.
- Early detection of elevated FPG levels, particularly in prediabetes, allows for lifestyle changes and interventions to prevent or delay the progression to full-blown diabetes.

Follow-Up Testing:

- If your FPG result is outside the normal range or if you have risk factors for diabetes, your healthcare provider may recommend additional tests, such as the Oral Glucose Tolerance Test (OGTT), to confirm the diagnosis.

Hemoglobin A1c (HbA1c)

Hemoglobin A1c (HbA1c) is a crucial blood test that measures the average level of glucose (sugar) in your blood over the past two to three months. It is an essential tool for the diagnosis and management of diabetes mellitus. HbA1c is also sometimes referred to as A1c, or glycated hemoglobin.

Purpose of the Hemoglobin A1c (HbA1c) Test:

- **Long-Term Blood Sugar Monitoring:** HbA1c provides a picture of your average blood sugar levels over a more extended period than other tests, which measure glucose at a specific moment in time. It helps healthcare providers assess how well blood sugar has been controlled over the past two to three months.

Test Procedure:

- The HbA1c test does not require fasting, and you can have it at any time of the day.
- A blood sample is drawn from a vein, usually in your arm.
- The collected blood is sent to a laboratory for analysis.

Interpretation of HbA1c Results:

- **Normal Range:** In individuals without diabetes, HbA1c levels are usually below 5.7%.
- **Prediabetes:** HbA1c levels between 5.7% and 6.4% indicate prediabetes, which is a higher-than-normal blood sugar level but not yet diabetes.
- **Diabetes:** A diagnosis of diabetes is typically made if your HbA1c level is 6.5% or higher on two separate tests.

Advantages of HbA1c:

- **Long-Term Monitoring:** Unlike fasting plasma glucose or oral glucose tolerance tests, HbA1c provides a more comprehensive view of blood sugar control over time.
- **Less Affected by Daily Fluctuations:** It is less influenced by daily variations in diet, physical activity, or stress.

Implications:

- Elevated HbA1c levels indicate that blood sugar control may not be adequate, which can increase the risk of diabetes-related complications such as heart disease, kidney problems, and nerve damage.
- Lowering HbA1c through lifestyle changes, medication, or insulin therapy is often a primary goal in diabetes management.

Frequency of Testing:

- The frequency of HbA1c testing varies depending on individual circumstances and the stage of diabetes management. For well-controlled diabetes, it may be tested every 3–6 months. In less stable conditions, it may be tested more frequently.

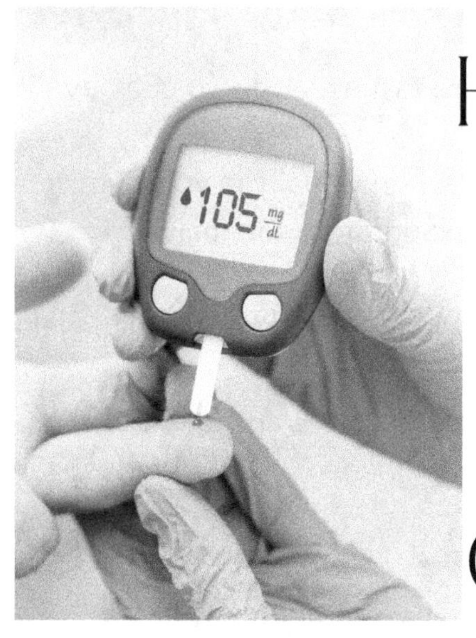

HOW DOES THE BODY MANAGE EXCESS GLUCOSE?

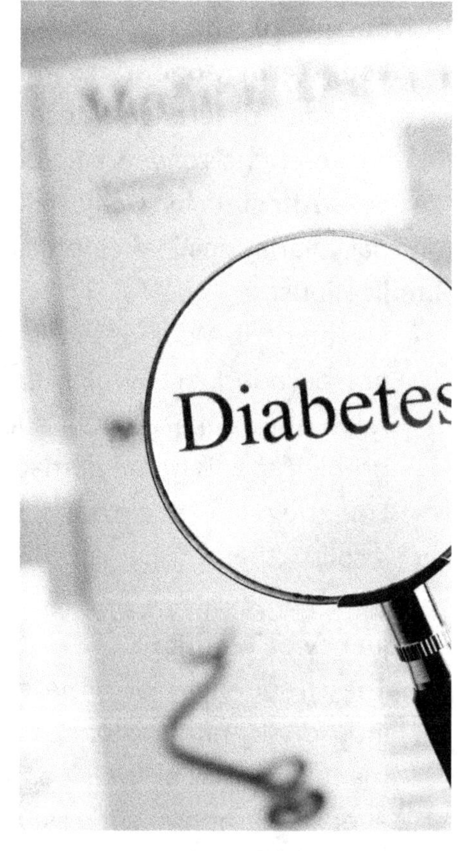

Now, when there is an excess amount of glucose in the body, the body will have to store up this glucose as it cannot remain in the bloodstream. In the following paragraph, we are going to break down the several mechanisms that the body could use to manage excess glucose. In order to have an effective understanding of how the body stores glucose, it is important to know the definitions of certain terms used in describing these processes

Glycogenesis: Glycogenesis is a complex biological process through which the body converts glucose into glycogen. This process primarily occurs in the liver and muscles and plays a crucial role in regulating blood sugar levels by storing up glucose in a readily available and accessible form. During periods of increased energy demand, such as physical activity or fasting, glycogen can be broken down into glucose through a process called glycogenolysis.

Lipogenesis: Lipogenesis is the biological process by which the body creates new fat molecules, called **triglycerides**, from various sources, including dietary carbohydrates, proteins, and excess calories. This process occurs mainly in the liver and adipose tissues. Lipogenesis is an essential part of energy storage, as excess calories that are not immediately needed for energy are converted into fat for storage in adipose tissue. This stored fat can later be used for energy when the body requires it. Lipogenesis is regulated by various hormones and enzymes in response to dietary and metabolic signals.

Note

Triglycerides: Triglycerides are a compact form of glucose stored as fat. The conversion of glucose into fatty acids and triglycerides allows for the efficient packing of a large amount of glucose into a relatively small space. Triglycerides act as a long-term energy reserve, providing a source of fuel during times of fasting or energy deficits.

Storage Sites

Certain organs in the body are targets for glucose storage. Some of these organs include the liver, adipose tissues, and skeletal muscles.

Liver: The liver is the second-largest organ in the human body and is responsible for several homeostatic processes in the body one of which is converting and storing glucose as glycogen in a process called glycogenesis. The body equally stores glucose in our skeletal muscles in the form of glycogen, and again, glycogenesis is the process of glycogen formation.

Adipose tissues: Adipose tissues, also known as fat tissues, are a type of connective tissue in the body. The cells that make up adipose tissues are called adipocytes. Adipocytes are specialized in storing fat and glucose, but it is important to note that for glucose to be stored in these adipocytes, it must be converted into fatty acids and undergo a series of processes before it can be stored in the adipose tissues. Adipose tissues are present in various parts of your body, including beneath the skin (subcutaneous fat), surrounding internal organs (visceral fat), and even within the inner spaces of bones (bone marrow adipose tissue), but they are most abundant in the abdomen, buttocks, and thighs.

When excess glucose circulates throughout the body and gets to the adipose tissues, it is converted into fatty acids in a process called lipogenesis. When the body wants to store up glucose for a longer period of time, it then combines the glucose that has been converted to fatty acids with *glycerol* to form triglycerides. When the glucose is in the form of triglycerides, the body now proceeds to store it into adipocytes, and this is that extra skin we see as we gain weight.

Note

Glycerol, also known as glycerin, is a simple organic compound with a sweet taste. It is a key component of triglycerides. Glycerol plays a crucial role in various biological processes and is involved in the structure and metabolism of fats.

Skeletal muscles: Fats can be stored in the muscles in the form of intramuscular triglycerides (IMTGs) or intramyocellular lipids

(IMCLs). While adipose tissue (fat tissue) is the primary site of fat storage in the body, very small amounts of fat can also accumulate within the muscle cells.

Note:

The fats discussed in this stage are the excess glucose molecules that the body has converted to fats through the process of lipogenesis.

Intramuscular triglycerides (IMTGs)

Intramuscular triglycerides (IMTGs) refer to the storage of triglycerides within the muscle cells. IMTGs serve as a local energy source for muscle metabolism during exercise or periods of increased energy demand.

Intramyocellular lipids (IMCL)

Intramyocellular lipids (IMCL) are a broader term that encompasses various types of **lipids** stored within the muscle cells, including triglycerides, phospholipids, and cholesterol esters. IMCL represents the overall lipid content within the muscle tissue.

While small amounts of IMTGs are considered normal and can provide energy during exercise, excessive accumulation of intramuscular lipids has been associated with conditions like insulin resistance, impaired glucose metabolism, and reduced muscle insulin sensitivity.

Note

Lipids are a broad group of organic molecules that include fats, oils, waxes, and certain vitamins (like vitamins A, D, E, and K). In organic solvents, they dissolve, but not in water. Lipids serve various functions in the body, such as storing energy, providing insulation, forming cell membranes, and serving as signaling molecules.

RISK FACTORS OF TYPE 2 DIABETES AND PREDIABETES

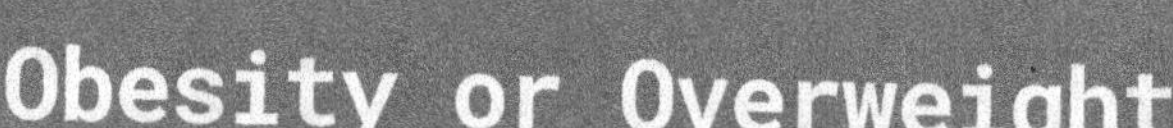

When considering obesity, we often tend to associate it with excessive eating and inadequate physical activity, and while this assumption is partly true, our understanding of its causes has evolved over time. It is now recognized that insulin plays a significant role in promoting weight gain.

Obesity or Overweight

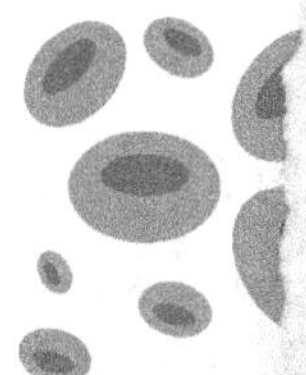

Both individuals with type 1 and type 2 diabetes who require insulin, as well as their doctors, are aware of this fact, which has been supported by numerous research studies.

This realization indicates that hormones such as insulin and **cortisol** are largely responsible for regulating body weight. It may seem logical to attribute weight gain to calorie intake, but it is not solely determined by the quantity of calories consumed. When excessive calories are ingested, the body compensates by burning them off, while insufficient calorie intake results in fewer calories being burned.

So, when we consume meals rich in carbohydrates, these carbs are broken down to glucose in the small intestine and absorbed into the bloodstream. Insulin is secreted in response to the rise in blood glucose and tells the liver to convert this glucose into fat. The conversion of glucose to fats by the liver causes more weight gain than just eating foods high in calories. This tells us that insulin is one of the main driving factors for weight gain, which can result in obesity. In people suffering from obesity, the cells of the body become saturated with glucose, requiring greater amounts of insulin to store glucose in these glucose-saturated cells. This process eventually leads to insulin resistance, which underlies the development of type 2 diabetes. Obesity, therefore, stems from a hormonal imbalance in fat regulation, particularly elevated levels of insulin. Increased insulin levels lead to greater glucose uptake by cells and a higher rate of conversion of glucose into fats.

2. **Intake of fattening carbohydrates**

Fattening carbohydrates refer to carbohydrate-rich foods that are more likely to contribute to weight gain and obesity when consumed in excess. These carbohydrates are often highly processed and have a **high glycemic index**, meaning they cause a rapid spike in blood sugar levels.

Note:

The glycemic index (GI) is a scale that measures how quickly carbohydrates in food raise blood sugar levels compared to pure glucose. Foods with a high glycemic index cause a rapid spike in blood sugar levels, while foods with a low glycemic index cause a slower, more gradual increase. Foods with a lower GI are often preferred because they provide more sustained energy and may help regulate blood sugar levels.

As these fattening carbohydrates are consumed over a long period of time, the insulin levels in our body rise, and this rise leads to obesity, which later on leads to insulin resistance and type 2 diabetes.

Some fattening carbohydrate meals include

1. Bread and everything made with flour
2. Cereals and milk puddings
3. All sweets
4. Foods containing a lot of sugar
5. Potatoes and white root vegetables

3. Physical inactivity

Another important factor that could lead to type 2 diabetes and prediabetes is physical inactivity. Whenever we exercise, our muscles convert the glycogen back to glucose in a process called glycogenolysis and use it for energy, but as the exercise continues, the glycogen stores become depleted. The fat stored in adipose tissue is mobilized and transported to the muscle cells, where it undergoes breakdown **(lipolysis)** to release fatty acids, which are then further broken down through a process called "beta-oxidation" to produce energy.

Note:

Just like glucose, fatty acids can also be used by the cells for the production of energy. In fact, fatty acids are a major source of energy, especially for tissues like muscle and the heart. When the body needs energy, fatty acids can be broken down through *a process called beta-oxidation to produce **ATP**, the body's primary energy currency. This process is particularly important during times of prolonged exercise or fasting when glucose stores become depleted.*

This process induces the body to lose some weight as the previously stored fats are burned up, and as this happens, the cells in the body gradually become more and more sensitive to insulin. This increase in sensitivity arises from the fact that glucose in the cells is converted to energy during this intense physical activity, causing our cells to regain their ability to absorb glucose efficiently.

In the case of an individual who doesn't exercise, the processes of fat breakdown mentioned above will not occur, and over time, a lot of glucose accumulates in the cells, leading to insulin resistance and eventually type 2 diabetes.

Note:

***Lipolysis** is the breakdown of triglycerides (fat molecules) stored in adipose tissue into their constituent components, glycerol and fatty acids. These fatty acids can then be transported to cells throughout the body, where they are further broken down through a process called "beta-oxidation" to produce energy in the form of adenosine triphosphate (ATP). Lipolysis typically occurs when the body needs additional energy, such as during periods of fasting, exercise, or when the intake of calories is lower than the energy expenditure. It is an essential metabolic process that helps to provide a source of energy when glucose (sugar) levels are low, as in between meals or during prolonged physical activity.*

***Glycogenolysis** is the biological process by which glycogen, a complex carbohydrate stored in the liver and muscles, is broken down into its simpler glucose units. This process releases glucose into the bloodstream, where it can be used to* *provide energy to cells and tissues throughout the body. Glycogenolysis is an important mechanism that helps regulate blood glucose levels and ensures a constant supply of glucose is available for various bodily functions, especially during periods of increased energy demand. It plays a crucial role in maintaining blood sugar homeostasis and providing a quick source of energy when needed.*

Potential Complication of Type 2 Diabetes

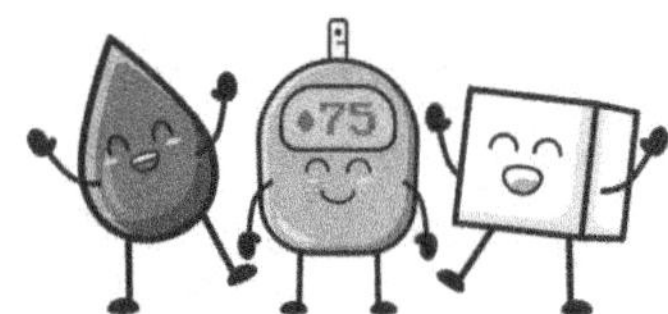

N. KEHSENI MARKBRON

Throughout our exploration, we have witnessed the body's continuous efforts to maintain low and balanced levels of glucose in the bloodstream.

Potential Complications of Type 2 Diabetes

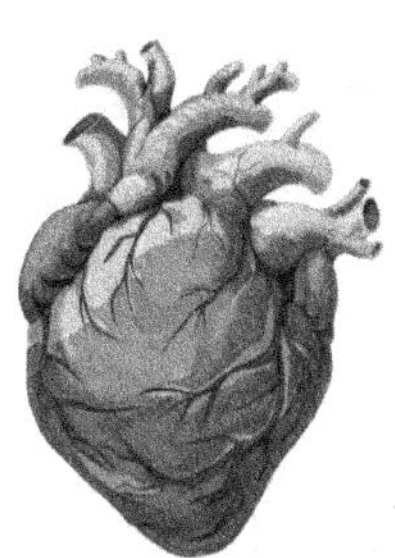

Throughout our exploration, we have witnessed the body's continuous efforts to maintain low and balanced levels of glucose in the bloodstream. We have equally seen how it has developed mechanisms to store excess glucose, telling us that the body doesn't seem to like something about glucose sitting in the bloodstream in very large amounts. Let's note that the normal fasting blood glucose range for individuals without diabetes, considered to be in a healthy or normal state, is between 70 and 99 mg/dL (3.9 to 5.5 mmol/L). This leads us to the question: Why does the body go through the trouble of mobilizing glucose to cells and organs? Can't all of that glucose simply remain in the bloodstream?

It is very important to understand that the reason why the body mobilizes glucose to the cells and organs is not just for energy production and storage but, more importantly, because of the several complications that arise when excess glucose circulates in the blood for extended periods. These complications can significantly worsen a diabetic patient's health condition.

In this chapter, we want to look at why the body doesn't like too much glucose circulating in the blood stream, focus on what happens when too much glucose accumulates in the blood stream over prolonged periods, and equally look at what happens when type 2 diabetes is poorly managed.

When an excess amount of glucose circulates in the blood stream for long periods, it damages our blood vessels, and this damage is what brings about the different complications we see in diabetic patients. Blood vessels are a tubular network of tissues that permit blood to circulate throughout our body. Blood vessels can be divided into small vessels (microvascular) and large vessels (macrovascular).

There are some major destructive processes that occur in the blood vessels of diabetic patients as a result of prolonged exposure to high glucose, and these processes occurring in the blood vessels are the underlying mechanisms behind the macrovascular and microvascular complications we see in diabetes patients. It is important to understand this process caused by glucose in the blood vessels because it will help us equally understand the different complications associated with type 2 diabetes.

First, we are going to look at the major destruction that occurs in the macrovessel (large blood vessels) before we talk about the destruction that occurs in the microvessel (small blood vessel). Below is the major destructive process occurring in the macrovessel.

Underlying mechanisms in macrovascular complications
   1. **Endothelial Dysfunction**
Endothelial dysfunction is a condition that affects the inner lining of blood vessels, known as the endothelium. The endothelium plays a crucial role in the contraction and relaxation of blood vessels, regulates blood clotting by releasing substances that promote or inhibit clot formation, produces nitric oxide, a molecule that helps blood vessels relax, promotes proper blood flow, and much more

When glucose sits in the blood vessel for too long, it causes the endothelium to become dysfunctional, impairing some of its major functions, such as blood clot regulation. Endothelial dysfunction is the major underlying mechanism behind macrovascular destruction. It is important to discuss this mechanism so as to have a better understanding of the macrovascular complications of diabetes. Let's now look at how endothelial dysfunction occurs in depth.

Many factors can cause endothelial dysfunction in a diabetic patient, but let's discuss a few.

Note

When we inhale air, the oxygen from the air gets into our lungs and diffuses into the blood stream. These oxygen molecules are transported from the blood stream to the various cells of our body by the red blood cells. When these oxygen molecules get into our cells, they react with glucose in a chain reaction to produce energy, a process called oxidation, so oxygen basically kickstarts the conversion of glucose to energy. Any time this reaction between oxygen and glucose occurs, it produces a byproduct, which is carbon dioxide. This carbon dioxide is transported back to the lungs by the red blood cells (RBC), and it leaves the body when we exhale. It is important to know that the accumulation of excess carbon dioxide in the blood can be harmful and lead to respiratory acidosis, causing a range of complications.

- **Formation of Reactive Oxygen Species (ROS)**

When there is an excess amount of glucose in our blood, the endothelial cells will take it up just like other cells do, but the interesting thing here is that these endothelial cells don't need insulin to take up glucose. As excess glucose gets into the endothelial cells, they react with oxygen (that you breathe) to produce a lot of energy through oxidation. One of the byproducts formed in the reaction between this excess amount of glucose and oxygen in the endothelial cell is *reactive oxygen species*. Reactive oxygen species (ROS) are highly reactive molecules that contain oxygen, and they are produced as natural byproducts of various cellular processes, one of which is the conversion of excess glucose into energy within the cell.

When ROS is formed in the endothelium, it leads to a cascade of events *(hyperglycemia-induced endothelial dysfunction)*, which causes inflammation of the endothelial cells, causing endothelial dysfunction, which is characterized by impaired barrier function and increased permeability of the endothelial layer.

Note:

Impaired barrier function: Impaired barrier function refers to a situation where the protective barrier, typically found in tissues like the endothelium (the inner lining of blood vessels), is not working correctly. This barrier is supposed to prevent unwanted substances from passing through, but when it's impaired, it becomes less effective at doing this job.

- **Dyslipidemia**

Individuals who consume a diet high in saturated fats, trans fats, and cholesterol and have little or no physical activity are at a heightened risk of developing dyslipidemia. Dyslipidemia is a disorder characterized by abnormal levels of lipids (fats) in the bloodstream, particularly elevated levels of **low-density lipoprotein cholesterol (LDL-C)** and **triglycerides,** which are all types of fats.

Now, one very interesting thing about this LDL-C is that it can also react with oxygen. and in the case of dyslipidemia, when an excess amount of LDL-C gets into the endothelial cells and reacts with oxygen. They also produce ROS as a byproduct, which in turn leads to **oxidative stress** that damages the endothelial cells.

Note

LDL (low-density lipoprotein): LDL, or low-density lipoprotein, is a type of lipoprotein—a combination of fat (lipid) and protein—that carries cholesterol in the bloodstream. Cholesterol is a waxy, fatty substance that is essential for building cell membranes and certain hormones but can be harmful when present in excess in the blood.

Oxidative stress: Oxidative stress is a condition that occurs when there is an imbalance between the production of reactive oxygen species (ROS) and the body's ability to detoxify them or repair the resulting damage. Reactive oxygen species are highly reactive molecules that contain oxygen and can cause damage to cells, proteins, and DNA. Normally, the body produces ROS as part of essential physiological processes, such as energy production and immune defense. However, excessive ROS production, often due to factors like environmental pollutants, UV radiation, a poor diet, or certain diseases, can overwhelm the body's antioxidant defenses. This leads to oxidative stress, which can result in cellular damage and dysfunction, inflammation, and an increased risk of various chronic diseases, including cardiovascular disease, neurodegenerative disorders, and cancer.

Macrovascular Complications

Now that we have established that endothelial dysfunction is the main underlying mechanism of macrovascular complications, let us proceed to discuss some of the macrovascular complications we see in diabetes and see how endothelial dysfunction brings about these different complications.

Atherosclerosis

Atherosclerosis is a condition characterized by the gradual buildup of plaque within the walls of arteries. We can think of a plaque as a fatty deposit within the inner layers of the arteries, and we should note here that arteries are macrovascular blood vessels, which are the larger blood vessels responsible for transporting blood and its content throughout the body.

Before we proceed to understand how atherosclerosis comes about in the macro vessel, let's have a brief study of the macro vessel and its different functions.

When we look at the arteries, they are tube-like in structure, and this tube-like structure is divided into layers.

The lumen: The lumen refers to the central open space or cavity within a tubular structure. That hollow space inside the vessel through which blood flows.

Tunica Intima: The tunica intima is the innermost layer of an artery, in direct contact with the blood flowing through it. It consists of three sublayers:

- **Endothelium:** This is a thin layer of specialized cells called endothelial cells. The endothelium provides a smooth surface for blood flow, helps regulate the dilation and constriction of the arteries (vascular tone), and maintains a barrier between the blood and the underlying layers.
- **Subendothelial Layer:** This layer lies beneath the endothelium and contains connective tissue with collagen fibers. It provides support and acts as scaffolding for the endothelium.
- **Internal Elastic Lamina:** This is a thin layer of elastic fibers located between the tunica intima and the tunica media. It

allows for flexibility and helps regulate the blood flow.

The tunica intima plays a crucial role in maintaining vascular integrity, regulating blood flow, and preventing the formation of blood clots.

Tunica Media: The tunica media is the middle layer of the artery and is composed of smooth muscle cells and elastic fibers. Its primary functions are:

- Contraction and Relaxation: The smooth muscle cells in the tunica media can contract or relax, allowing for changes in the diameter of the artery and regulation of blood flow and blood pressure.

- Elasticity: The elastic fibers within the tunica media allow arteries to expand and recoil, helping to maintain continuous blood flow and providing a buffer against sudden changes in blood pressure.

The tunica media is thicker in arteries compared to other blood vessels, reflecting its role in regulating blood flow and pressure.

- **Tunica Externa:** The tunic externa, also known as the tunica adventitia, is the outermost layer of an artery. It consists mainly of connective tissue, including collagen fibers. The functions of the tunica adventitia include:
- **Structural Support:** The collagen fibers provide strength and support to the artery, ensuring its shape and integrity.
- **Nourishment**: The tunica externa contains small blood vessels called vasa vasorum that supply nutrients and oxygen to the outer layers of the artery wall.
- **Anchoring:** The tunica adventitia anchors the artery to surrounding tissues, helping to maintain its position within the body.

PARTS OF THE ARTERY

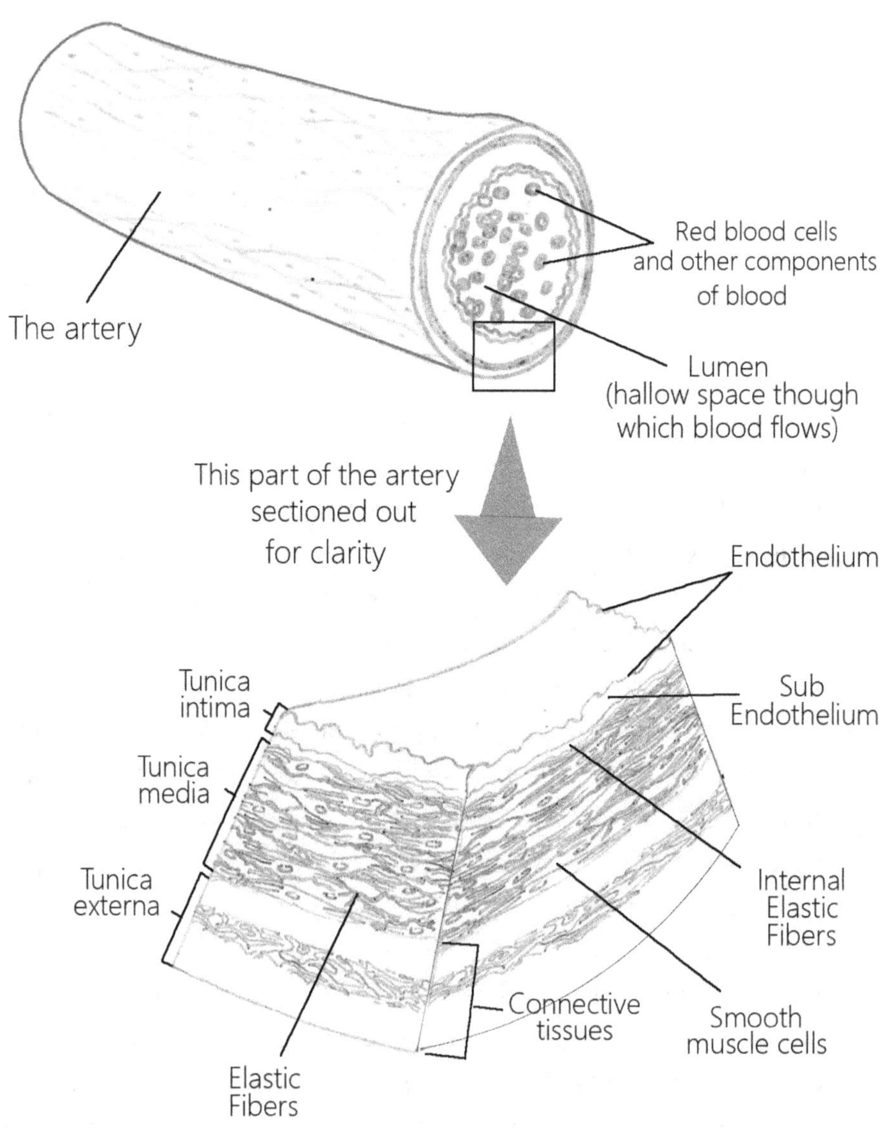

These three layers work together to facilitate the proper functioning of arteries, allowing for regulated blood flow, maintaining vascular tone, and ensuring structural integrity. The specific composition and characteristics of each layer can vary depending on the type and size of the artery.

Formation of Atherosclerosis

It is important to note that before the formation of an atherosclerosis plaque occurs in a diabetes patient, the endothelial layer of the arteries is already undergoing processes like the formation of reactive oxygen species due to the excessive amounts of glucose in the blood, which renders the endothelium dysfunctional. and so the dysfunctional endothelium eases the formation of atherosclerosis.

When there is an excess amount of low-density lipoprotein (LDL) in the blood stream, it will be taken up by these dysfunctional endothelial cells.

As this fat (LDL) gets into the endothelial cells, it reacts with the reactive oxygen species (previously produced in the endothelial layer by the reaction between excess glucose and oxygen), causing the low-density lipoprotein (LDL) to be oxidized. It is important to note that reactive oxygen species (ROS) are very reactive molecules; therefore, they readily react or bond with other molecules, such as low-density lipoprotein (LDL). The reaction between reactive oxygen species (ROS) and low-density lipoprotein (LDL) produces a byproduct known as *oxidized LDL.*

Note

A byproduct is essentially a residue produced from a reaction. You can compare byproducts to the carbon dioxide released from the exhaust pipe of a car when driving.

Oxidized LDL: Oxidized LDL (low-density lipoprotein) refers to LDL cholesterol particles that have undergone a chemical transformation known as oxidation. Oxidation is a process in which LDL cholesterol molecules are exposed to free radicals, or reactive oxygen species. This exposure can cause changes in the LDL particles, making them more reactive and potentially harmful to the cardiovascular system.

The problem with this oxidized LDL (byproduct) is that it is a pro-inflammatory substance with the ability to promote inflammation within the body. Another problem with low-density lipoprotein (LDL) getting into the endothelial cells is that once it is oxidized in the endothelial cells, it can no longer leave the endothelial cells, which means that it gets trapped there.
When this oxidation of LDL happens, the body will want to get rid of the byproduct (oxidized LDL) produced. Remember that the body expels carbon dioxide from the oxidation of glucose whenever we breathe out. But oxidized LDL is not a gas, so it cannot be expelled through breathing. So, as this oxidized LDL starts causing inflammation inside the endothelial tissues, the damaged tissues will release some chemicals into the bloodstream, and these chemicals are what signal the body defense system that there is a problem. So, the endothelial cells are then activated (opened up) to facilitate the entry of the body defense cells to come in and get rid of this oxidized LDL.

As the defense cells enter the endothelial cells, they engulf these oxidized LDL with the intention of destroying them. As they engulf these oxidized LDL, they become *foam cells* in the process, and as they become foam cells, they also get trapped beneath the endothelial layer. These foam cells are key to the formation of atherosclerosis. The main reason why foam cells are key in atherosclerosis is because foam cells release hormones that promote the migration of the smooth muscle cells from the Tunica Media (2nd layer of the artery) up into the Tunica Intima

(1st layer of the artery), causing the first layer to bulge up into the lumen and restricting the space for blood flow.

An increase in the proliferation of these smooth cells from the Tunica Media (2nd layer of the artery) into the Tunica Intima (1st layer of the artery) will lead to the hardening of the arteriosclerosis plaque. Over time, the foam cells will die, releasing their LDL content, and this cycle drives the growth of the plaque. It is important to remember that oxidized LDL is a pro-inflammatory substance.

Therefore, a combination of the dead foam cells and their LDL content, which is pro-inflammatory, together with the smooth muscle cells that have migrated into the Tunica Intima (1st layer of the artery) and all the defense cells that keep entering this first layer (endothelial cells) in order to evacuate the oxidized LDL will collectively drive the growth of the atherosclerosis plaque.A serious case of artheriosclerosis occurs when the artheriosclerosis plaque ruptures, spilling its contents into the lumen. When this happens, the body's natural response is to form a blood clot (**thrombus**) around the injured artery to prevent excessive bleeding. But this blood clot (thrombus) can further narrow the lumen, restricting the flow of blood, and a condition where blood flow is restricted by a blood clot is called **thrombosis.**

Note

Thrombosis is a medical condition where blood clots form within blood vessels, obstructing the normal flow of blood. These clots, known as thrombi, can occur in veins or arteries throughout the body. Thrombosis can lead to serious complications if the clot breaks loose and travels to vital organs such as the lungs, heart, or brain, causing conditions like pulmonary embolism, heart attack, or stroke

It's important to note that atherosclerosis is the most clinically significant and commonly discussed form of arteriosclerosis due to its association with cardiovascular diseases. However, understanding the broader concept of arteriosclerosis helps to recognize the various types of arterial changes that can occur in different contexts.

Note: *Arteriosclerosis is a broader term referring to the thickening and hardening of the arterial walls. While atherosclerosis is a specific type of arteriosclerosis characterized by the buildup of plaque in the arteries,*

FORMATION OF ATHEROSCLEROSIS

O_2 = **OXYGEN**

⬠ = **GLUCOSE**

◎ = **BLOOD CELL**

Co2 = **CARBON DIOXIDE**

1.)

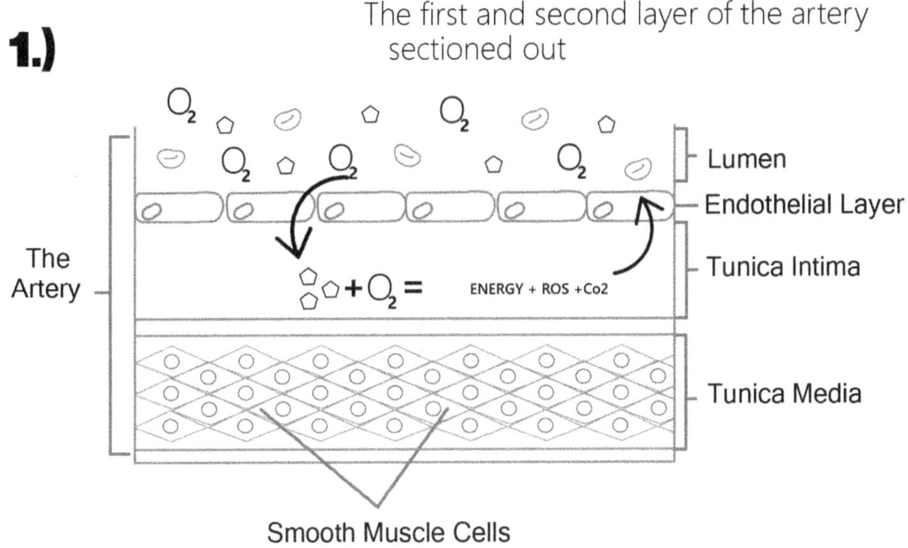

Excess glucose reacting with oxygen in the endothelial layer
to produce energy, reactive oxygen species and carbondioxide
as by-products. Carbondioxide diffuses out of the endothelial layer
to be expelled by the lungs.
This reaction between excess glucose and oxygen in the endothelial
layer triggers a cascade of events like inflammation which causes
the endothelial cells to become dysfunctional characterized by
impaired barrier function and increased permeability of the
endothelial layer.

FORMATION OF ATHEROSCLEROSIS

O_2 = **OXYGEN**

= **LOW DENSITY LIPO-PROTEIN (LDL)**

= **BLOOD CELL**

= **OXIDIZED LOW DENSITY LIPO-PROTEIN**

ROS = **REACTIVE OXYGEN SPECIE**

2.)

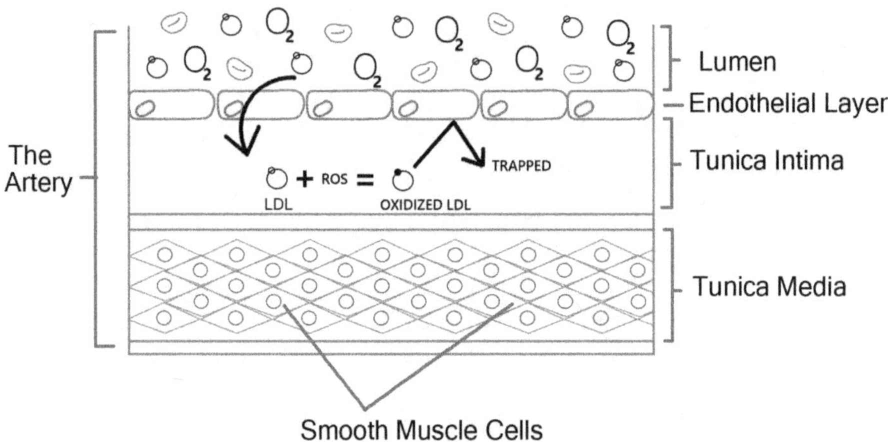

High amount of low density lipo-proteins in the blood a condition know as hyperlipidemia gets into the endothelial layer without the use of insulin.

Once in the endothelial layer, LDL reacts with reactive oxygen species previously formed from the reaction of excess glucose and oxygen Once LDL reacts with ROS, it produces a by product knows as Oxidized LDL. Oxidized LDL is proinflammatory and it kickstarts the formation of atherosclerosis.

FORMATION OF ATHEROSCLEROSIS

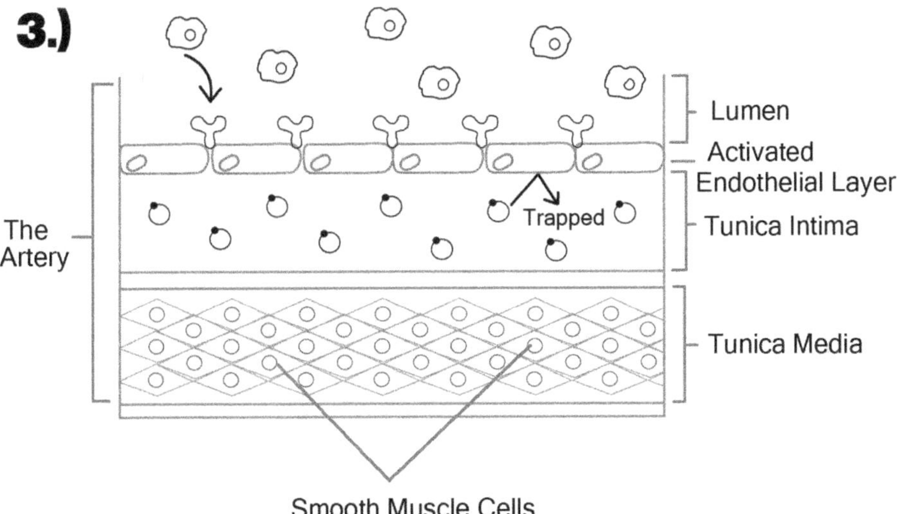

When Oxidized LDL gets trapped in the tunica intima, it starts causing inflammation. This causes the endothelial layer to release some chemical in the bloodsteam that signal the defense system that there is a problem. when the body defense cells get on site, the endothelial layer is activated and expresses adhesion molecules on its surface which facilitates the migration of the body's defense from the lumen into the tunica intima.

FORMATION OF ATHEROSCLEROSIS

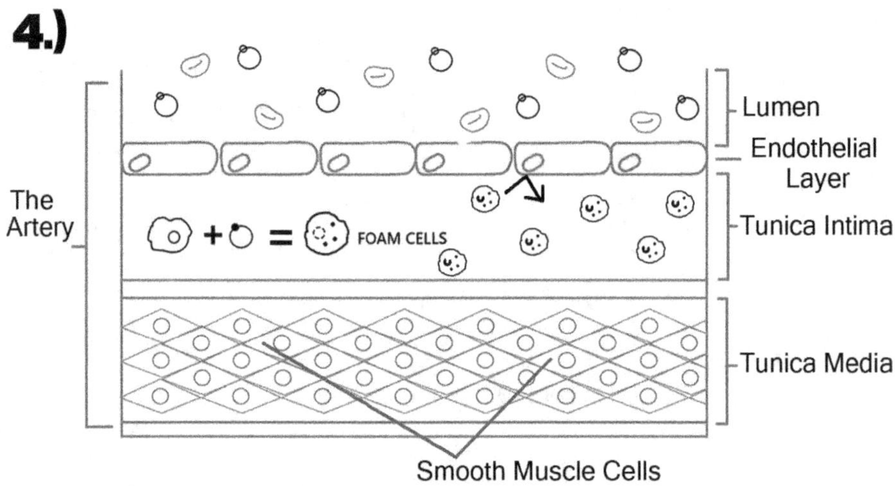

As the defense cells enter the endothelial layer, they engulf these oxidized LDL with the intention of destroying them. As they engulf these oxidized LDL, they become foam cells in the process, and as become foam cells,they also get trapped beneath the endothelial layer.

These foam cells are key to the formation of atherosclerosis.The main main reason why foam cells are key in atherosclerosis is because foam cells release hormones that promote the migration of the smooth muscle cells from the Tunica Media up into the Tunica Intima.

FORMATION OF ATHEROSCLEROSIS

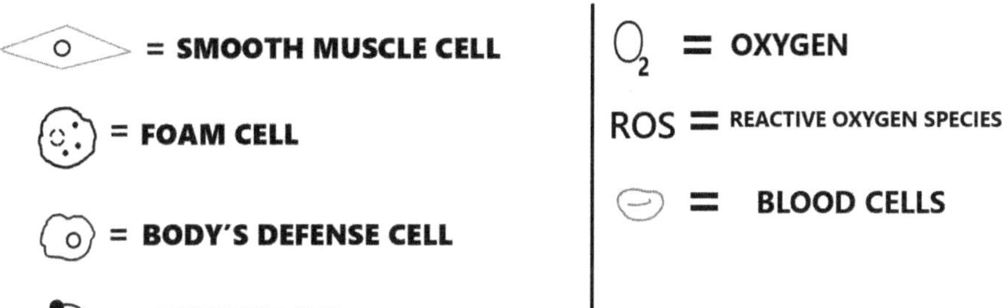

5.)

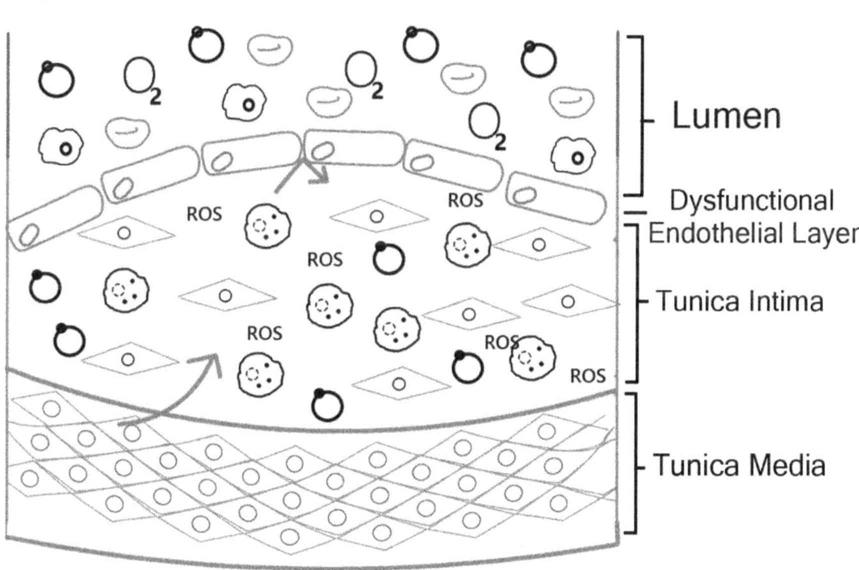

A combination of the dead foam cells and their LDL content, which is pro-inflammatory, together with the smooth muscle cells that have migrated into the Tunica Intima and all the defense cells that keep entering this first layer in order to evacuate the oxidized LDL will collectively drive the growth of the atherosclerosis plaque.

FORMATION OF ATHEROSCLEROSIS

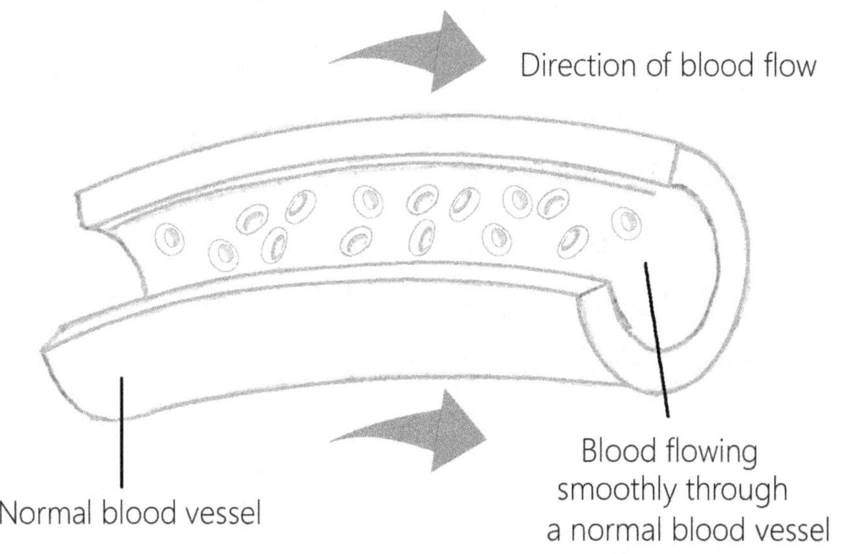

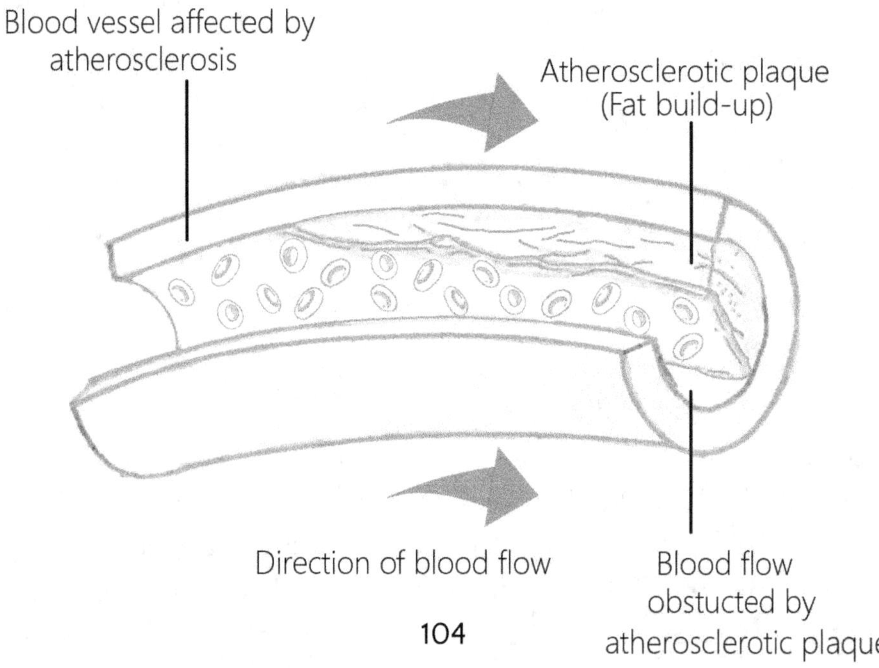

Coronary Artery Disease (CAD):

Coronary arteries are the blood vessels found around and inside your heart muscle, and their main function is to supply blood, oxygen, and nutrients to the heart, which enables the heart to function properly. Coronary artery disease (CAD) is a condition where the coronary arteries are narrowed by plaque formation or a blood clot commonly caused by artheriosclerosis, decreasing the supply of blood, oxygen, and nutrients to the heart, resulting in the death of the heart muscles, leading to heart attack, hypertension, and other heart problems. It is important to note that CAD is the most common type of heart disease and a leading cause of death worldwide.

- **Stroke**

A stroke, also known as a cerebrovascular accident (CVA), is a medical condition that occurs when the blood supply to a part of the brain is disrupted, leading to brain cell damage or death. Strokes can have serious consequences and are considered a medical emergency.

There are two main types of strokes:

1. **Ischemic Stroke:** This is the most common type of stroke, accounting for about 85% of all cases. Ischemic stroke occurs when a blood clot or plaque commonly formed by atheriosclerosis blocks or narrows an artery supplying blood to the brain. The blockage prevents adequate blood flow and oxygen from reaching the brain cells in the affected area.

2. **Hemorrhagic Stroke:** This type of stroke occurs when a blood vessel in the brain ruptures or leaks, leading to bleeding into or around the brain tissue. Hemorrhagic strokes can result from conditions such as high blood pressure (hypertension), aneurysms (weakened and bulging blood vessels), or arteriovenous malformations (AVMs), which are abnormal tangles of blood vessels.

Peripheral Artery Disease (PAD)

Peripheral Artery Disease (PAD), also known as peripheral vascular disease, is a condition that affects the arteries outside the heart and brain, most commonly the arteries in the legs. It is characterized by the narrowing or blockage of these arteries, leading to reduced blood flow to the limbs. PAD is primarily caused by atherosclerosis, the buildup of fatty deposits and plaque in the arterial walls.

The main risk factors for developing PAD include smoking, diabetes, high blood pressure, high cholesterol levels, obesity, older age, a family history of PAD or cardiovascular disease, and a sedentary lifestyle. These factors contribute to the development of atherosclerosis and the subsequent narrowing and hardening of the arteries.

Peripheral Artery Disease (PAD) can have several effects on the affected individual. These effects can vary depending on the severity of the condition and the extent of arterial blockage. Here are some common effects of PAD:

- **Claudication:** The most common symptom of PAD is intermittent claudication, which refers to pain, cramping, or fatigue in the muscles of the legs during physical activity. The pain typically subsides with rest. Claudication can limit a person's ability to walk or engage in physical activities, leading to reduced mobility and exercise intolerance.
- **Non-healing Wounds and Ulcers**: A chronic reduction in blood flow to the lower extremities can impair wound healing as the nutrients and hormones necessary to promote the healing of these wounds have been reduced due to the narrowing of the blood vessel by the atheriosclerosis plaque. Minor injuries or ulcers on the feet or legs may take longer to heal and have an increased risk of infection. Without proper treatment, these wounds can become chronic and may lead

Coronary artery disease (CAD)

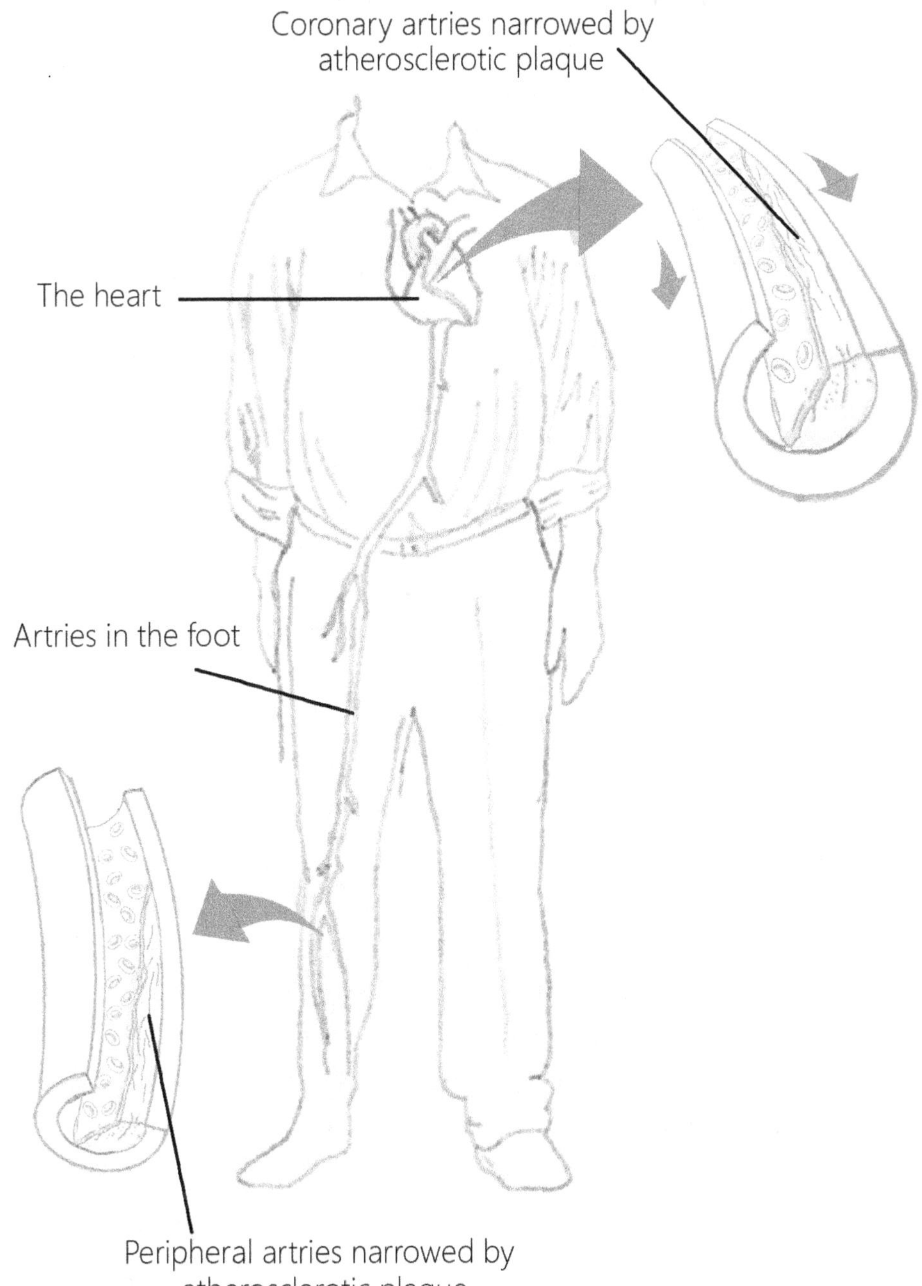

to the development of skin ulcers or gangrene.

- **Limb Ischemia:** Ischemia is a medical term that refers to an inadequate blood supply to a particular tissue, organ, or body part. It occurs when there is a reduction or complete blockage of blood flow through the arteries that supply oxygen and nutrients to the affected area. Severe cases of PAD can result in chronic tissue ischemia, even at rest. Inadequate blood flow to the affected limbs can cause pain, coldness, and discoloration. In severe cases, prolonged ischemia can lead to tissue damage, non-healing ulcers, and the potential for limb loss (amputation).

Microvascular Complications

Microvascular complications in the context of diabetes are long-term health problems that can occur in the micro vessels as a result of poorly controlled high blood glucose for extended periods. These complications occurring in the micro vessels primarily affect the eyes, kidneys, and nerves.

Underlying mechanisms in microvascular complications

In order to understand these microvascular complications, it is important to know the underlying mechanism behind them. There are numerous underlying mechanisms that contribute to the development of microvascular complications in diabetes. However, the following examples represent some of the most frequently encountered ones:

1. **Formation of Advanced Glycation End Products (AGEs):**

When an excess amount of glucose circulates in the blood stream for extended periods, it will react with the *hemoglobin* in red blood cells, proteins, and other components of the blood in a process called *glycation.* In the formation of early glycation products, glucose first reacts with fats such as LDL (low-density lipoproteins) and proteins. Over time, these early glycation products undergo a chain of chemical modifications, such as rearrangements and cross-linking, resulting in the formation of more complex and stable molecules known as AGEs (Advanced Glycation End Products).

Note:

Glycation: Glycation is a chemical reaction that occurs in the body when sugar molecules, such as glucose, bind to proteins or fats. One interesting thing is that this process occurs without the use of an enzyme (non-enzymatic) in a process called non-enzymatic glycosylation. The end result of glycation is the formation of molecules called advanced glycation end products (AGEs). AGEs can accumulate in various tissues in the body, including the skin, blood vessels, and organs.

Glycation and the subsequent formation of AGEs are a natural and ongoing process in the body, but excessive glycation can have detrimental effects. It is often associated with various health issues, particularly in the context of chronic conditions like diabetes. AGEs can contribute to inflammation, oxidative stress, and tissue damage, which may play a role in the development of complications related to diabetes.

When advanced glycation end products (AGEs) are formed, they will circulate around the body and form clogs in the blood vessels, especially the smaller blood vessels found in the kidney, eyes, and brain. This is so because advanced glycation end products (AGE) are very sticky compounds. When these clogs are formed, red blood cells and other types of blood cells will stick to these advanced glycation end products (AGEs), blocking the blood vessel and disrupting the smooth flow of blood.

These blocked blood vessels activate the body's defense system.

The body defense cells, in an attempt to destroy the clogs formed by these AGEs, will secrete inflammatory molecules called proinflammatory cytokines, which cause inflammation in the clogged-up area. These inflammations destroy the body's blood vessels, causing them to leak out their contents.

2.Impaired Nitric Oxide (NO) Production

Nitric oxide is a vital signaling molecule, meaning it communicates information within cells and between different cells. In physiological terms, signaling molecules like nitric oxide (NO) transmit messages that regulate various processes such as neurotransmission, immune response, and vascular function. Nitric oxide is produced by endothelial cells lining the blood vessels, and it plays a crucial role in the dilation and constriction of the blood vessels by:

- **Vasodilation**: One of the primary functions of nitric oxide is to promote vasodilation, the relaxation and widening of blood vessels. When released by endothelial cells, nitric oxide diffuses into the underlying smooth muscle cells of the blood vessel, where it stimulates the production of **cyclic guanosine monophosphate (cGMP).** cGMP relaxes the smooth muscle cells, causing vasodilation and allowing for increased blood flow. This process helps regulate blood pressure, improve circulation, and ensure adequate oxygen and nutrient delivery to tissues.
- **Anti-inflammatory Effects**: Nitric oxide possesses anti-inflammatory properties. It can inhibit the expression and activity of pro-inflammatory molecules, such as adhesion molecules and cytokines, in endothelial cells and immune cells. By reducing inflammation, nitric oxide helps maintain the integrity and function of the blood vessel wall and limits the recruitment and activation of immune cells within the vessel.

- **Inhibition of Platelet Aggregation**: Nitric oxide helps prevent the excessive aggregation of **platelets**, which are responsible for blood clot formation. It inhibits platelet activation, adhesion, and aggregation by interfering with platelet signaling pathways and reducing platelet reactivity. This antiplatelet effect of nitric oxide helps maintain normal blood flow and prevents the formation of unwanted blood clots.

When you have elevated glucose for extended periods, it will get into the endothelial cells and cause endothelial dysfunction. When this happens, the production of nitric oxide by the endothelial cells becomes impaired, leading to a decrease in the production of nitric oxide. When there is an absence of nitric oxide, you experience complications such as:

- **Impaired Vasodilation**: One of the primary functions of NO is to promote vasodilation, relaxing the smooth muscles in blood vessels and increasing their diameter. Impaired NO production leads to reduced vasodilation capacity, resulting in impaired regulation of blood flow, increased vascular resistance, and elevated blood pressure.
- **Inflammation and Immune Dysfunction:** NO (Nitric Oxide) has anti-inflammatory properties and helps regulate immune responses within blood vessels. Impaired NO production disrupts the balance between pro-inflammatory and anti-inflammatory factors, leading to increased inflammation and altered immune cell activity. This chronic inflammation contributes to the progression of vascular damage and the onset of microangiopathy.

Note

Microangiopathy refers to a disease affecting the small blood vessels, particularly the arterioles and capillaries.

- **Platelet Aggregation and Thrombosis:** NO (Nitric Oxide) inhibits platelet activation and aggregation, preventing the formation of blood clots. Inadequate NO production disrupts this antiplatelet effect, leading to increased platelet reactivity and aggregation. This increases the risk of thrombosis, the formation of blood clots within blood vessels, which can obstruct blood flow and lead to further complications such as a heart attack or stroke.

3.Sorbitol Formation and Osmotic Stress

Sorbitol Formation:

Another mechanism underlying the microvascular complications we see in diabetic patients is sorbitol formation.

When you have elevated levels of glucose for extended periods, this glucose will be converted into a sugar alcohol known as sorbitol with the help of the enzyme **aldose reductase** found in the cells. There are many reasons behind the conversion of glucose to sorbitol in the cell, but let's highlight a few.

Note:

Enzyme aldose reductase: Aldose reductase is an enzyme that plays a role in the metabolism of sugars, specifically in the processing of glucose and other simple sugars (aldoses). Its primary function is to convert glucose into another sugar called sorbitol through a chemical reaction known as reduction.

- **Cellular energy storage**

The conversion of glucose to sorbitol serves as a means for cells to handle excess glucose. In certain tissues, such as the liver and adipose tissue, glucose can be converted to sorbitol as a means of storage. Sorbitol can be further metabolized to generate energy when needed. However, this energy storage function of sorbitol is relatively minor compared to other metabolic pathways, such as glycogen storage.

- **Regulation of Osmotic Balance**

One of the key functions of sorbitol in the cells is to manage osmotic pressure within the cells. It does so by drawing water into the cell to avoid dehydration, thus making sorbitol a *humectant*. Sorbitol draws water primarily from the extracellular space, meaning it draws water from the surrounding fluid outside the cells. When sorbitol accumulates within cells, it creates an osmotic gradient, which leads to the movement of water from the extracellular space into the cells to equalize the solute (glucose) concentrations. By increasing the intracellular osmolarity through sorbitol accumulation, water flows into the cell to maintain equilibrium, preventing excessive water loss or cellular dehydration. This osmotic regulation helps cells maintain their proper shape, volume, and function.

Note

Sorbitol has a water retention property that helps the cell maintain its osmotic pressure, shape, volume, and cellular function. A molecule that has a water retention property is often referred to as a humectant. Humectants are substances that attract and retain moisture from the surrounding environment.

Omotic stress

In a person suffering from diabetes, when there is excess glucose in the bloodstream, this glucose is converted to sorbitol. One thing about sorbitol is that it is not easily used up or metabolized by the cell like glucose, and due to this, sorbitol keeps accumulating in the cell. Since sorbitol is a humectant, it increases the osmotic pressure of the cell, causing water molecules to keep entering the cell from extracellular space. This causes the cell to swell up, and now the continuous swelling of the cell as a result of increased osmotic pressure is what we refer to as osmotic stress. And this is very dangerous because it can cause cellular damage, causing the organ in which this cell experiences this continuous osmotic pressure to be dysfunctional.

The continuous accumulation of sorbitol in the cells, leading to osmotic stress, is one of the major underlying mechanisms happening in the blood vessels of diabetic patients, which causes some of the complications we see in diabetes.

Hypertension:

Another intriguing mechanism that is an underlying mechanism of the microvascular complications we see in diabetes is hypertension, or high blood pressure. If you are a high blood pressure patient suffering from diabetes, it can increase your risk of getting some microvascular complications associated with diabetes, as hypertension causes serious damage to the blood vessels.

Hypertension exerts increased force on the walls of blood vessels throughout the body, including the small blood vessels known as capillaries. Over time, this heightened pressure can cause several detrimental effects on these delicate vessels, ultimately contributing to microvascular complications. Some of the processes caused by hypertension on these smaller blood vessels (capillaries) include:

1. **Endothelial Damage**: The endothelium, which is the thin layer of cells lining the interior surface of blood vessels, can be severely injured due to prolonged hypertension disrupting their normal functions. This damage is caused by the increased pressure on the endothelial cells, which can lead to inflammation and dysfunction of the endothelium, impairing its ability to regulate blood flow and maintain vascular tone.
2. **Vascular Remodeling**: Chronic hypertension can trigger remodeling processes in the blood vessel walls, including

thickening and stiffening of the vessels to overcome the high pressure the blood exerts on them and prevent the vessel from bursting. These structural changes can narrow the diameter of capillaries, reducing blood flow to vital organs and tissues.

Types Of Microvascular Complications

Now that we have gained an understanding of the underlying mechanisms, we can delve deeper into examining the microvascular complications.

Diabetic Retinopathy

Diabetic retinopathy is a common microvascular complication of diabetes that affects the eyes. It occurs as a result of damage to the blood vessels in the *retina*, the light-sensitive tissue at the back of the eye. Diabetic retinopathy is a progressive condition that can lead to vision loss and even blindness if left untreated.

The development of diabetic retinopathy is closely associated with chronic and poorly managed hyperglycemia (high blood sugar levels) over an extended period of time. Prolonged exposure to high blood sugar leads to processes such as the formation of sorbitol, the formation of advanced glycated end products (AGEs), etc. that damage the small blood vessels in the retina.

In order to have a good understanding of diabetic retinopathy's pathophysiology (functional changes that occur in the body as a result of disease or injury), it is important to understand some key parts of the eye and their functions.

THE EYE AND ITS PARTS

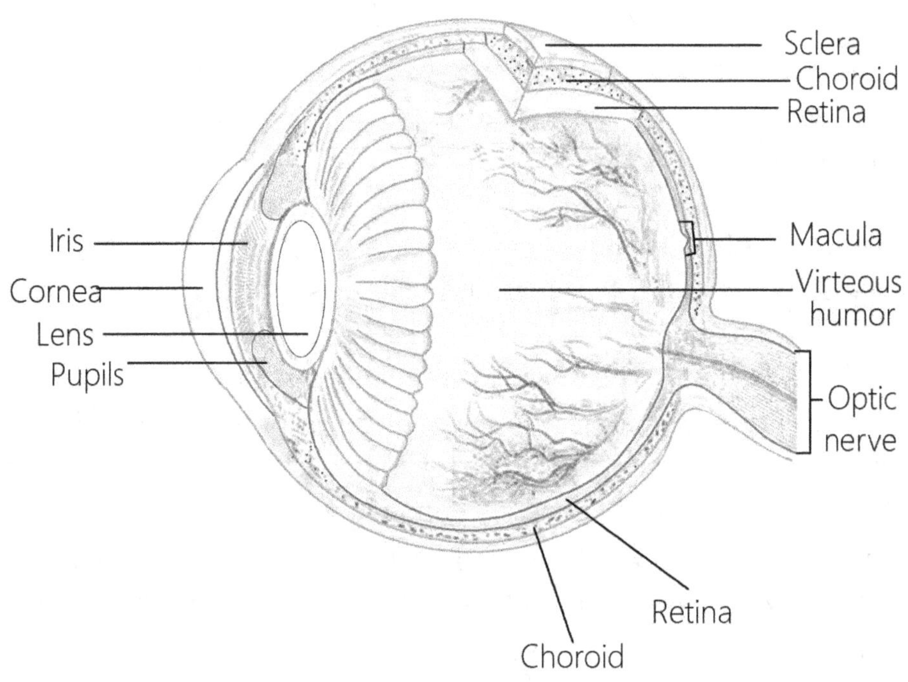

Here is a list of the different parts of the eye that are necessary for explaining diabetic retinopathy:

1. **Cornea**: The transparent front surface of the eye that acts as a protective barrier and helps focus light onto the retina.
2. **Iris**: The coloured part of the eye that, by adjusting the pupil size, controls the quantity of light entering the eye.
3. **Pupil**: The black circular opening in the center of the iris that lets light into the eye.
4. **Lens**: A clear structure located behind the iris that helps to further focus light onto the retina.
5. **Retina**: The innermost layer of the eye that contains light-sensitive cells (rods and cones) and plays a central role in the vision process.
6. **Macula**: A small area in the center of the retina responsible for sharp, detailed vision and color perception.
7. **Optic Nerve**: The bundle of nerve fibers that carries visual information from the retina to the brain.
8. **Vitreous Humor**: The clear, gel-like substance that fills the space between the lens and the retina.
9. **Blood Vessels**: The network of blood vessels that supply the retina with oxygen and nutrients. This includes the central retinal artery and vein.
10. **Choroid**: A layer of blood vessels that lies between the retina and the sclera (the white part of the eye) and supplies blood to the outer layers of the retina.

Now that we have a very basic general orientation to the eye, let's use this knowledge of the eye to discuss diabetic retinopathy. Diabetic retinopathy can be classified into three stages:

1. **Early Stages of Diabetic Retinopathy**

The first stage of diabetic retinopathy is called "diabetes without retinopathy" because, in this stage, individuals with diabetes do not exhibit any clinical signs or symptoms of retinopathy when their eyes are examined. This stage is primarily characterized by the absence of visible retinal changes or abnormalities, despite the presence of diabetes. And so, long before someone with diabetes develops vision problems, the underlying hyperglycemia or high blood sugar levels in their blood start causing damage to the *pericytes* within the retina.

Pericytes are specialized cells found within the tiny blood vessels, known as capillaries, throughout the human body. They play a vital role in maintaining the health and functionality of these blood vessels. Chronic exposure to high blood sugar levels can damage the pericytes in retinal capillaries. Damage to these pericytes is believed to be caused by the inability of these cells to properly metabolize glucose due to insulin resistance, and the damage is caused by some processes that occur when glucose sits in the bloodstream for too long.

Some of these processes include the formation of sorbitol, which results in osmotic stress and slowly progresses into cellular damage; the formation of AGEs; oxidative stress; and much more. This damage weakens the capillary walls, making them prone to leakage. Retinal pericytes surround the retinal vasculature, and they're very important for helping regulate blood flow throughout the retina.

This damage to the retinal pericytes is the earliest stage of diabetic retinopathy, and it's likely present in many, if not most, individuals who have had diabetes for at least a few years.

However, this damage is only detectable under a microscope, and therefore the retina on ophthalmology or on an eye exam looks normal. So, in the early course of diabetes, individuals will not necessarily have visual disturbances or signs of disease on an exam. However, this does not necessarily mean that the damage is not occurring; it's just not detectable.

2. **Non-proliferative diabetic retinopathy (NPDR)**

In non-proliferative or pre-proliferative diabetic retinopathy, we observe that the critical role of retinal pericytes in regulating blood flow across the retinal vessels is altered. When these pericytes sustain damage, it leads to a weakening of the capillary walls, and since the pericytes are damaged, they lose their ability to regulate blood flow in the retinal vessels, leading to increased blood flow in these vessels.

These damaged capillaries facilitate the development of microaneurysms, which are localized expansions of the weakened vessel walls. These aneurysms form within the microvasculature of the retina and manifest as small red dots dispersed unpredictably throughout the retina. They are often detected during ophthalmologic examinations.

Note:

Microaneurysms: Microaneurysms are tiny, localized bulges or outpouchings that occur in the smallest blood vessels, particularly capillaries, in the body. In the context of diabetic retinopathy, they are focal dilations of weakened vessel walls found in the microvasculature of the retina. These microaneurysms are a hallmark of diabetic retinopathy and are often among the initial clinical signs of the condition. While they can occur in various parts of the body, they are of particular concern when they develop in the retina, as they can lead to vision problems and are a critical feature in the assessment and diagnosis of diabetic retinopathy.

These microaneurysms, though somewhat challenging to observe, appear as dots within the retina. These dots are typically the earliest clinical indication of diabetic retinopathy. Nonetheless, the non-proliferative or pre-proliferative diabetic retinopathy stage is marked not only by these microaneurysms.

It also involves damage to the retinal capillaries (blood vessels), leading to enhanced vascular permeability. In simple terms, it means that the capillaries become leaky, enabling large molecules, such as proteins and lipids (fat molecules) usually contained within these microblood vessels, to escape into the retinal tissue. When this happens, the body doesn't have a natural mechanism for reabsorbing these leaked substances back into the body. Consequently, proteins and lipids that escape from these damaged capillaries become trapped within the retinal tissue.

This leakiness and its consequences can be detected during a dilated eye exam, which features numerous microhemorrhages or microaneurysms in the retina. These proteins and fats that have leaked out of the blood vessel are seen as white-yellow flecks.

These clinical findings of proteins and fats in the retinal tissues distinctly characterize the second stage, namely, non-proliferative or pre-proliferative diabetic retinopathy. This stage, however, may or may not present noticeable symptoms. And this stage usually begins about 15 to 25 years after an individual's initial diabetes diagnosis and may persist for several years before progressing further.

3. **Proliferative diabetic retinopathy (PDR)**:

Proliferative diabetic retinopathy may not always show symptoms, but this is quite rare. In most cases, individuals who reach this stage of diabetic retinopathy will typically experience at least blurred vision or notice the presence of floaters.

As the name suggests, proliferative diabetic retinopathy is characterized by the growth of new blood vessels within the retina. This happens because the microvascular damage that occurs in the earlier stages of diabetic retinopathy (pericyte damage, development of microaneurysms, and vascular permeability) destroys the blood vessel in the retina, which will result in reduced blood supply to the retina, leading to a condition called ischemia. Ischemia refers to a lack of oxygen supply to the retinal cells. It is important to note that blood transports oxygen and nutrients throughout the body, and where there is reduced blood flow, there is less oxygen and nutrient supply. In order to compensate for this lack of oxygen and nutrient supply, the retina produces a growth factor known as **VEGF**, which stands for *vascular endothelial growth factor.* VEGF, as its name implies, stimulates the formation of new blood vessels within the retina in a process called neovascularization. However, in diabetic retinopathy, these new blood vessels are very weak and prone to leakage.

Note

Neovascularization refers to the abnormal formation of new blood vessels, often in response to conditions like ischemia (restricted blood supply) or hypoxia (low oxygen levels) in tissues. This process can occur in various parts of the body and is particularly significant in the context of diabetic retinopathy, where abnormal blood vessel growth in the retina can lead to vision problems and even blindness.

As more VEGF is produced by the retina as a result of reduced blood flow over time, this will result in the development of numerous new blood vessels within the retina. The development of these new blood vessels can be observed during a dilated eye examination, and they present themselves as new, irregularly shaped blood vessels within the retina.

Unfortunately, when diabetic retinopathy advances to this third stage and becomes proliferative, the clinical progression becomes unpredictable and can be quite severe, potentially leading to vision-threatening complications like **vitreous hemorrhage** or retinal detachment.

DIABETIC RETINOPATHY

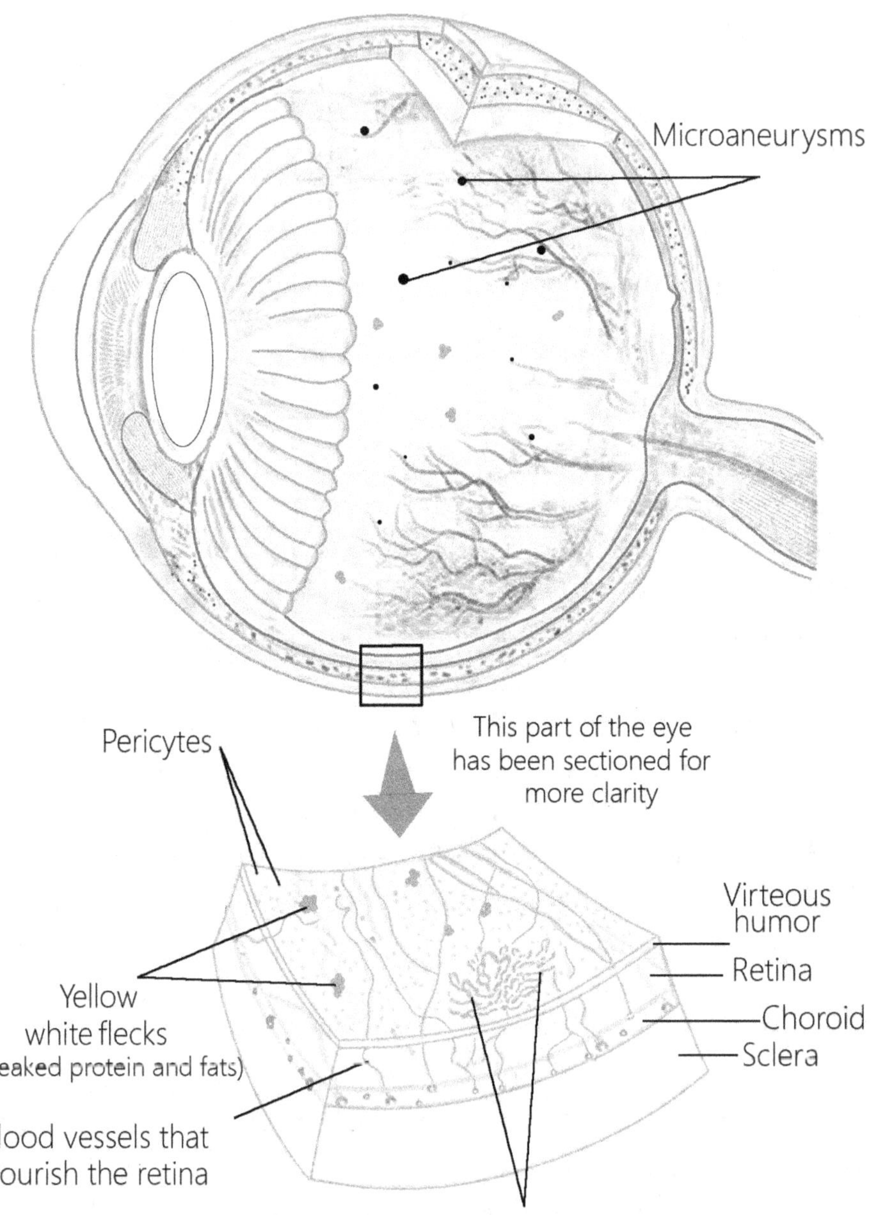

Abnormal formation of new and weak blood vessels
in response to conditions like ischemia

Note

Vitreous hemorrhage: *A vitreous hemorrhage is a medical condition characterized by bleeding into the vitreous humor, which is the gel-like substance that fills the center of the eye. This bleeding can occur due to various reasons, such as trauma, diabetic retinopathy, or other retinal disorders. It can lead to symptoms like sudden vision loss, floaters (spots or specks in the vision), or blurred vision, and may require medical intervention to address the underlying cause and manage the bleeding.*

Retinal detachment: *Retinal detachment is a serious eye condition where the retina, the thin layer of tissue at the back of the eye that detects light, separates from its normal position. This detachment can occur due to various reasons, such as injury, age-related changes, or other eye diseases. Symptoms of retinal detachment may include sudden flashes of light, floaters (spots or specks in the vision), and a curtain-like shadow over the field of vision. Retinal detachment requires prompt medical attention to prevent permanent vision loss, typically through surgical intervention to reattach the retina to the back of the eye.*

Diabetic Nephropathy

One of the significant long-term complications of diabetes mellitus is a condition referred to as diabetic nephropathy. Breaking down the term into "nephro" and "pathy" reveals that it literally denotes kidney disease secondary to diabetes. This condition is quite prevalent, impacting approximately 20% to 40% of individuals with diabetes, encompassing both type I and type II diabetes. In this chapter, we aim to discuss this diabetic complication in depth, revealing the different processes that make diabetic nephropathy so fatal.

In order to have a clear understanding of this disease, it is important to have detailed knowledge of how the kidney functions.

THE KIDNEY

The Medulla

Renal vein

(carries filtered blood
away from the kidney
to the rest of the body)

Renal artery
(carries blood into the
kidneys for filtration)

Uretha
(carries filtrate (urine) to the bladder
for excretion)

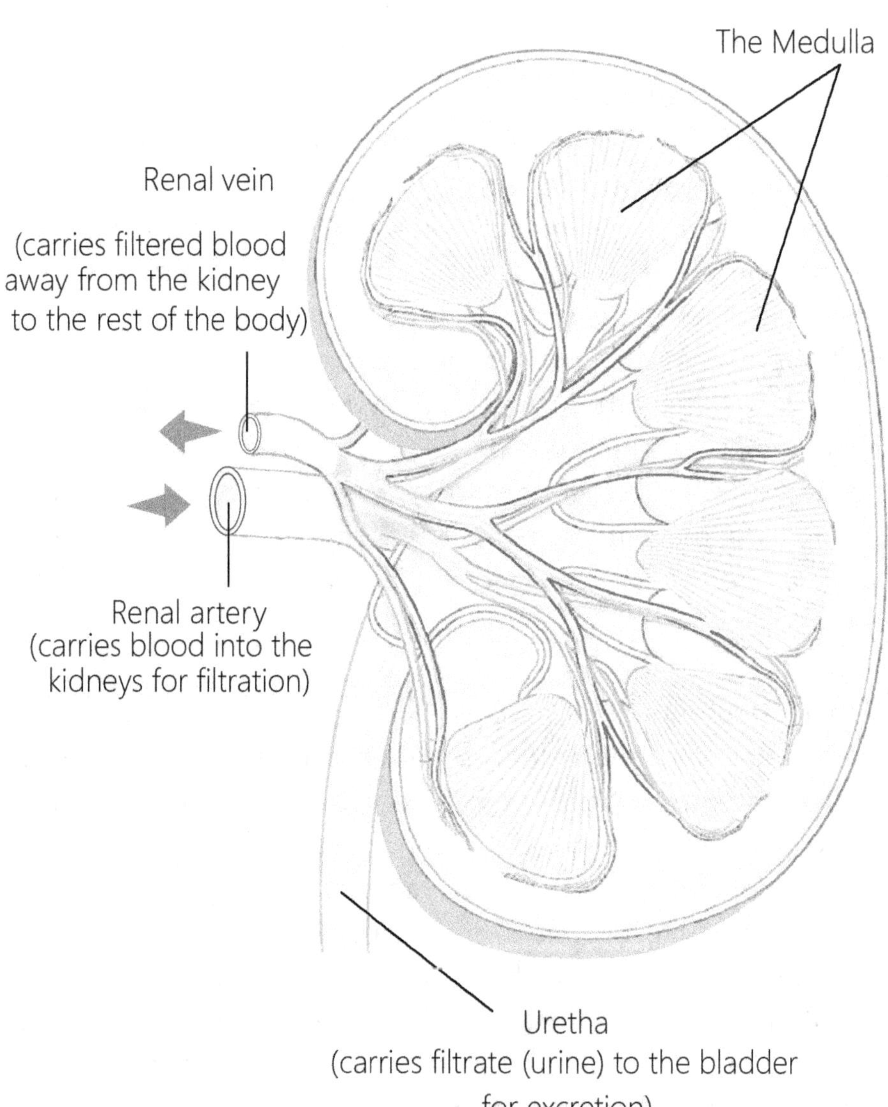

THE MEDULLA OF THE KIDNEY

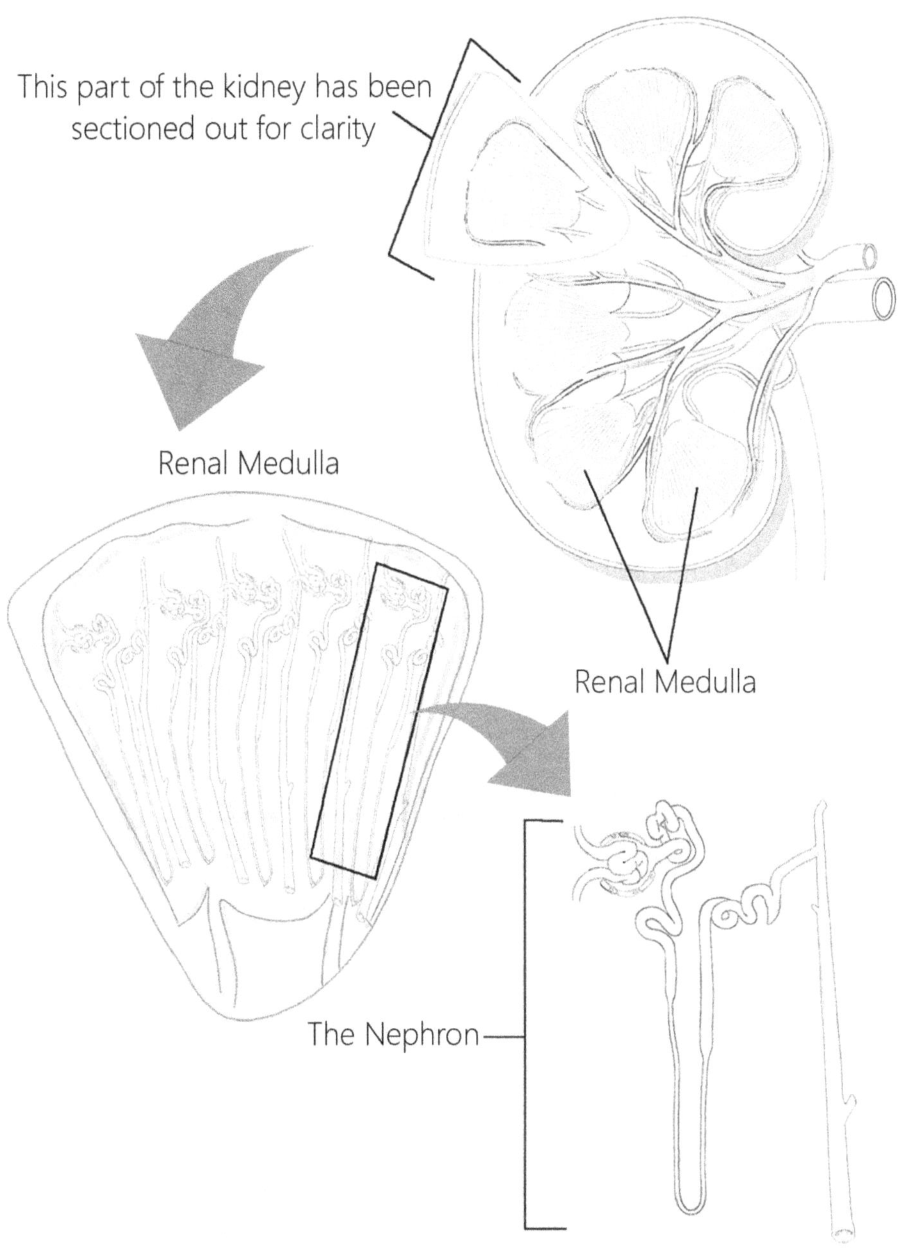

THE NEPHRON

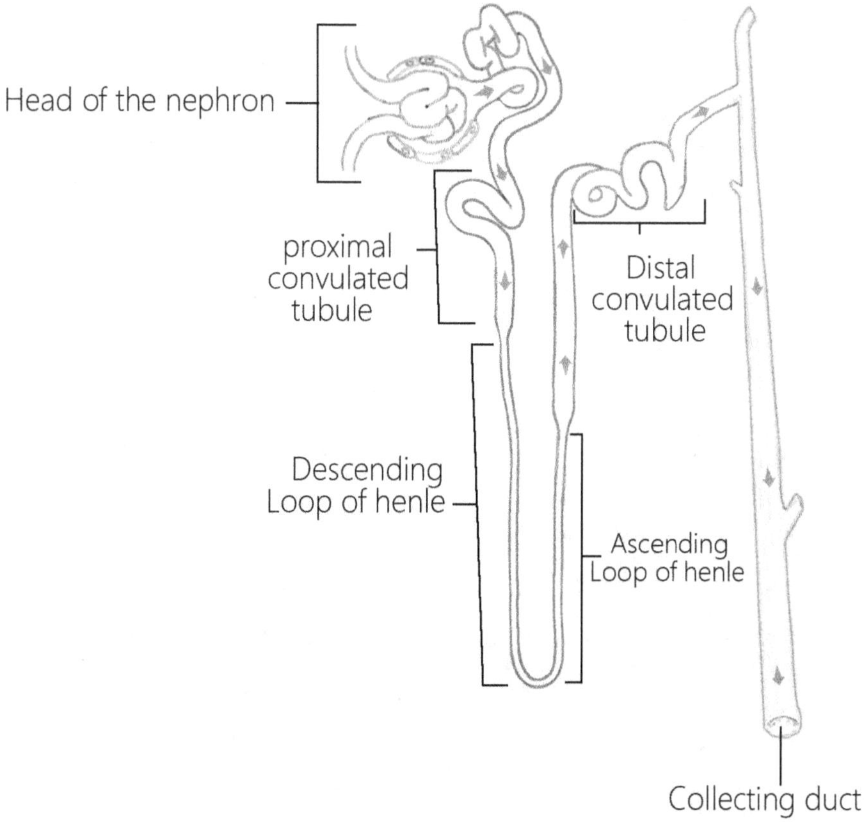

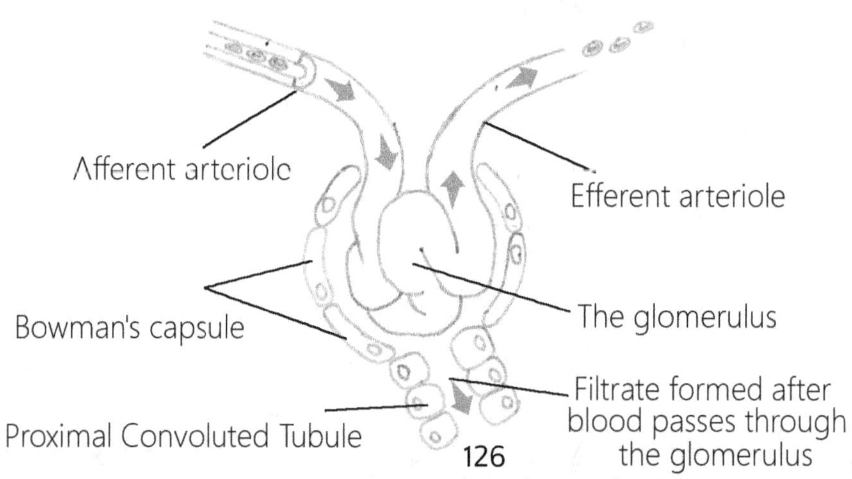

HEAD OF THE NEPHRON

CROSS SECTION OF THE NEPHRON

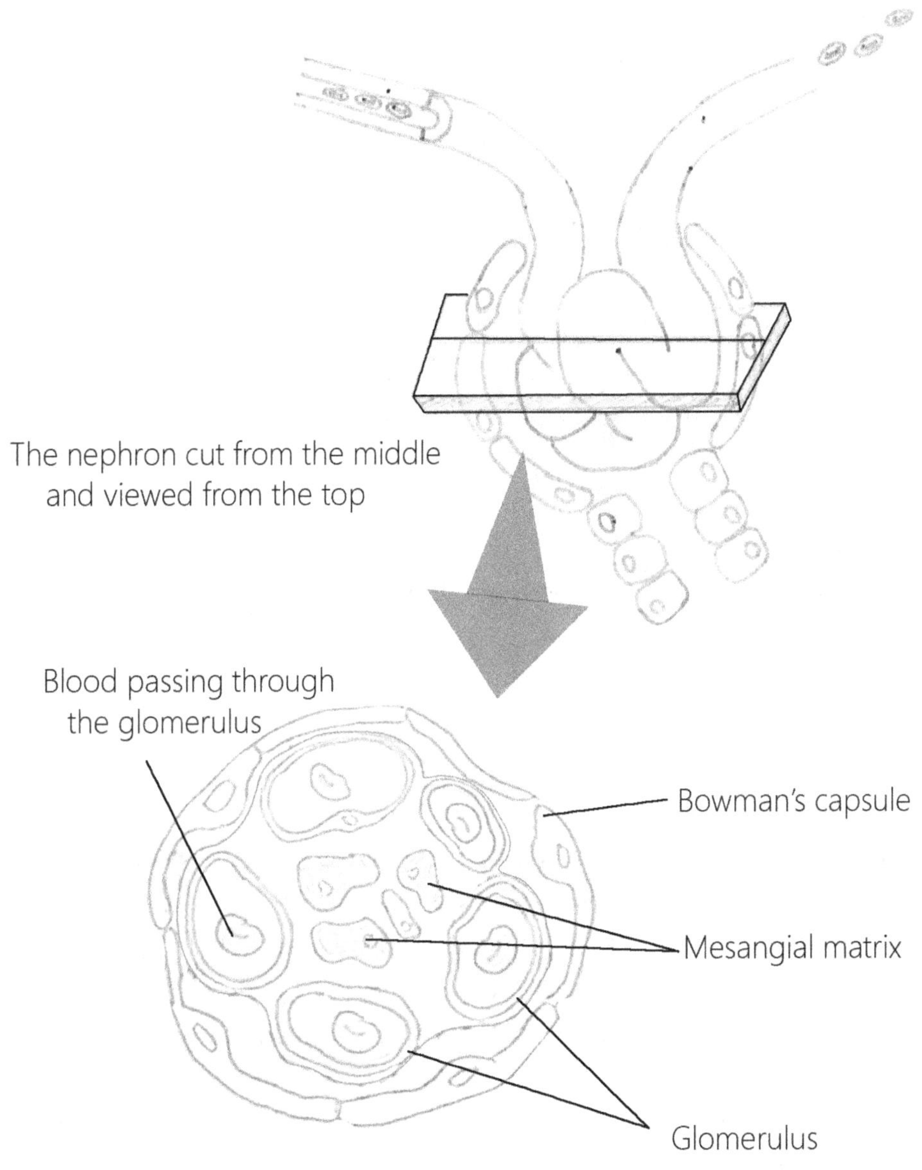

View of the nephron from
the top. this view reveals
the inner components of the
nehron affected by diabetes

The kidney is a vital organ in the human body that plays a crucial role in maintaining overall health. The functional unit of the kidney is the nephron, which is responsible for the filtration of blood and the formation of urine. Each kidney contains approximately one million nephrons, and they are essential for maintaining the body's internal environment by regulating water and electrolyte balance and removing waste products.

Humans typically have two kidneys, one on each side of the spine, below the ribcage. Some of the main functions of the kidneys include filtration of blood, blood pressure regulation, erythropoiesis regulation, acid–base balance, and toxin excretion. But in the context of diabetic nephropathy, we want to focus mainly on blood filtration, blood pressure regulation, and toxin excretion.

Parts of the Kidney

1. Parts of the Kidney Responsible for Filtration

One major function of the kidney is the filtration of blood, and below are some of the parts of the kidney responsible for this process of filtration.

The nephron

The nephron is the functional unit of the kidney; that is, the nephron is a distinct component within the kidney that performs a specific function or set of related functions. The nephron is responsible for filtering and processing blood to form urine. Each kidney contains thousands of nephrons, and they play a crucial role in maintaining the body's fluid and electrolyte balance. The nephron is divided into two sections, which consist of a *renal corpuscle* and a **renal tubule.**

Glomerulus:
The glomerulus is a tiny, ball-shaped cluster of blood vessels located on the nephron in the kidney. It is an integral part of the nephron. The glomerulus plays a crucial role in the initial stage of urine formation by filtering blood, allowing water, electrolytes, and small molecules to pass through while retaining larger substances like proteins and blood cells.

The glomerulus is surrounded by a structure called Bowman's capsule, and together they form the renal corpuscle. As blood flows through the glomerulus, a filtrate is produced by the selective passage of substances based on their size and charge. This filtrate then undergoes further processing in the renal tubules to eventually form urine, which is excreted from the body. The efficient functioning of the glomerulus is vital for maintaining proper fluid and electrolyte balance in the body.

The mesangium
The mesangium is a structural component within the glomerulus. The glomerulus consists of a network of tiny blood vessels, and the mesangium is located between and around these vessels.
Specifically, the mesangium is made up of mesangial cells and a ***mesangial matrix***. Mesangial cells are specialized cells found in the renal corpuscle, and they provide structural support to the capillaries in the glomerulus. These cells also have contractile properties, influencing the blood flow within the glomerulus.
The mesangial matrix is a gel-like substance that surrounds the mesangial cells. It contributes to the structural integrity of the glomerulus and is involved in regulating the filtration process. The mesangium plays a role in modulating the surface area available for filtration and in maintaining the permeability of the glomerular capillaries.

Bowman's capsule

Bowman's capsule is a key component of the renal corpuscle, which is part of the nephron in the kidney. The Bowman's capsule surrounds and encapsulates the glomerulus.

The primary function of Bowman's capsule is to collect the filtrate that is produced as blood passes through the glomerulus. During filtration, water, electrolytes, and small molecules move from the blood into Bowman's capsule, forming the initial filtrate. This filtrate then continues its journey through the renal tubule, where additional processes such as reabsorption and secretion take place to refine and concentrate it into urine. Together, the glomerulus and Bowman's capsule make up the renal corpuscle.

The Afferent Arteriole

The afferent arteriole is a small blood vessel that carries blood into the glomerulus, which is a cluster of capillaries (small blood vessels) responsible for blood filtration in the kidney. Structurally, it arises from a larger blood vessel branching off the renal artery and leading directly into the glomerulus.

The primary function of the afferent arteriole is to deliver blood to the glomerulus at a controlled rate. This steady influx of blood ensures that the glomerulus maintains the appropriate pressure needed for effective filtration. The pressure is crucial for forcing small molecules such as waste products, electrolytes, and water out of the blood and into the kidney tubules, where urine formation begins.

The diameter of the afferent arteriole can be adjusted to regulate blood flow into the glomerulus. This regulation is critical for maintaining a stable glomerular filtration rate (GFR), which ensures that waste products are effectively removed from the blood without excessive loss of essential substances. For example, constriction of the afferent arteriole decreases blood flow into the glomerulus, reducing filtration, while dilation increases blood flow and filtration.

Changes in the diameter of the afferent arteriole can equally have significant effects on kidney function. For instance, constriction of the afferent arteriole may occur in response to decreased blood volume or blood pressure, helping to maintain systemic blood pressure by redirecting blood flow to vital organs. Conversely, dilation of the afferent arteriole increases blood flow and filtration, which may be necessary to increase urine production and eliminate excess fluid from the body.

The Efferent Arteriole

The blood vessel leaving the glomerulus is called the efferent arteriole. It arises from the network of capillaries (small blood vessels) within the glomerulus and carries blood away from the glomerulus.

Blood entering the glomerulus through the afferent arteriole is under high pressure, which is necessary for the filtration of waste products and excess substances from the blood. The efferent arteriole regulates this pressure by controlling the rate at which blood leaves the glomerulus. This regulation is vital for maintaining the glomerular filtration rate (GFR), which ensures that essential substances are filtered while retaining necessary components in the bloodstream.

The efferent arteriole plays a crucial role in regulating blood flow within the kidney. By constricting or dilating, it can adjust the resistance to blood flow, thereby influencing the pressure within the glomerulus. Constriction of the efferent arteriole leads to increased pressure within the glomerulus, enhancing filtration, while dilation decreases pressure, reducing filtration.

Changes in the diameter of the efferent arteriole have significant effects on renal function. For example, constriction of the efferent arteriole can increase glomerular pressure and filtration, which may be necessary in certain physiological states. Conversely, dilation of the efferent arteriole reduces glomerular pressure and filtration, which can occur under conditions where preservation of fluid volume or blood pressure is essential.

How does filtration occur in the kidney?
The kidneys' three-layered filtration system is a highly specialized process crucial for maintaining fluid and electrolyte balance in the body. This intricate system primarily involves the afferent arteriole, **vascular endothelium**, glomerular basement membrane, and visceral epithelium (podocytes).

The process begins as blood enters the glomerulus through the afferent arteriole. In the glomerulus, the vascular endothelium, composed of fenestrated endothelial cells, forms the first layer of the filtration system. These specialized cells have small pores or fenestrations that allow small molecules such as water, electrolytes, and waste products to pass through, but they retain larger components like blood cells and proteins.

The second layer is the **glomerular basement membrane,** a dense extracellular matrix that acts as a selective barrier. It prevents the passage of larger particles, ensuring that essential components remain in the bloodstream. This membrane serves as a key component in determining the size and charge selectivity of the filtration process in the glomerulus.

The final layer is the **visceral epithelium,** consisting of podocytes. Podocytes are unique, branched cells with foot-like extensions that wrap around the capillaries of the glomerulus. These extensions form filtration slits, creating a highly selective barrier that allows only small molecules to pass through. Podocytes actively contribute to the regulation of filtration by adjusting the size of the filtration slits.

As the blood is being filtered through this 3-layer filtration system in the glomerulus, this filtrate goes down the Bowman's capsule and into the renal tubules for reabsorption.

2. Parts for Reabsorption and Secretion

When the filtrate from the glomerulus gets into the renal tubules, it still contains some important components of blood, and as such, it cannot just be expelled out of the body without these components being reabsorbed. Now let's look at the different parts of the kidney responsible for the reabsorption of these components from this glomerular filtrate.

Renal tubules:

Renal tubules are small, tube-like structures found within the nephron of the kidney that play a crucial role in the reabsorption and secretion processes that occur during urine formation.

The renal tubules extend from the Bowman's capsule, which surrounds the glomerulus, and are organized into three main segments: the proximal convoluted tubule (PCT), the loop of Henle, and the distal convoluted tubule (DCT). These tubules work in coordination to modify the composition of the filtrate, adjusting the levels of water, electrolytes, and other solutes based on the body's needs.

Proximal Convoluted Tubule (PCT):

The Proximal Convoluted Tubule (PCT) is a segment of the renal tubule within the nephron. It is located immediately after the Bowman's capsule, and it plays a crucial role in the process of urine formation.

The primary function of the proximal convoluted tubule is

reabsorption, It is responsible for the reabsorption of the majority of filtered substances from the glomerular filtrate back into the bloodstream. This includes essential molecules such as glucose, amino acids, ions, and the majority of filtered water. As the filtrate passes through the PCT, these substances are actively or passively transported across the tubular cells and reabsorbed into the *peritubular capillaries* surrounding the tubules.

Loop of Henle

The Loop of Henle is a U-shaped portion of the renal tubule within the nephron. This tubular structure is essential for the concentration and dilution of urine.

The Loop of Henle is divided into three parts: the descending limb, the thin ascending limb, and the thick ascending limb. Each segment has distinct functions in the reabsorption and concentration of urine.

1. **Descending Limb:** The descending limb allows water to pass out of the tubule into the surrounding interstitial fluid, increasing the concentration of the filtrate as it descends deeper into the medulla of the kidney.
2. **Thin Ascending Limb:** The thin ascending limb is permeable to ions, allowing the passive diffusion of sodium and chloride out of the tubule. This contributes to an increasing concentration of the surrounding interstitial fluid.
3. **Thick Ascending Limb:** The thick ascending limb actively transports sodium, potassium, and chloride ions out of the tubule. This segment is impermeable to water, so no water is reabsorbed here. The net effect is the dilution of the filtrate.

The Distal Convoluted Tubule (DCT)

The Distal Convoluted Tubule (DCT) is a segment of the renal tubule within the nephron. The DCT is located after the Loop of Henle and is responsible for further processing the filtrate that has passed through the earlier parts of the nephron.

The primary functions of the distal convoluted tubule include fine-tuning the reabsorption of electrolytes and water and participating in the secretion of certain substances into the filtrate. Unlike the Proximal Convoluted Tubule (PCT), the DCT plays a more selective role in reabsorption, responding to hormonal signals and the body's specific needs.

The DCT regulates the balance of ions, such as sodium, potassium, and calcium, based on the body's requirements. It is influenced by hormones such as aldosterone, which promotes the reabsorption of sodium and water, and parathyroid hormone, which enhances calcium reabsorption. Additionally, the DCT plays a role in maintaining the body's acid–base balance by secreting hydrogen ions and reabsorbing bicarbonate.

Peritubular capillaries

Peritubular capillaries are small blood vessels that surround and closely associate with the **renal tubules** in the nephron. These capillaries play a vital role in the reabsorption and secretion processes that occur during the formation of urine.

The peritubular capillaries arise from the efferent arterioles that exit the glomerulus, which is the initial filtering component of the nephron. As the filtrate flows through the renal tubules, the peritubular capillaries closely follow the path of the tubules, allowing for efficient exchange of substances between the blood and the renal tubular cells.

1. **Reabsorption:** Essential substances, such as water, glucose, ions, and other solutes, that are reabsorbed from the renal tubules are transported into the peritubular capillaries. This process helps to return important molecules to the bloodstream and maintain the body's homeostasis.
2. **Secretion:** Substances that need to be eliminated from the

body, such as certain waste products and excess ions, are actively transported from the peritubular capillaries into the renal tubules. This contributes to the formation of urine.

The peritubular capillaries, along with the vasa recta (specialized capillaries associated with the Loop of Henle), create a network that allows for the exchange of substances to occur along the entire length of the renal tubules. This close association is essential for the kidneys' role in regulating the composition of the blood and forming urine.

3. **Parts of the Kidney Responsible for Excretion:**

Below are the parts of the kidney responsible for the excretion of waste from the kidney after the blood has been filtered.

- **The ureter**

The ureter is a muscular tube that serves as a duct for urine, transporting it from the kidneys to the urinary bladder. Each human kidney has one ureter, and the ureters play a crucial role in the excretory system by facilitating the passage of urine from the kidneys, where it is produced, to the urinary bladder, where it is stored until it is expelled from the body during urination.

Underlying factors contributing to diabetic nephropathy

In the context of diabetes, a lot of processes can contribute to diabetic nephropathy, but let's discuss two main factors.

1. **Hypertension**

Now that we have an overview of how the kidney functions, let us proceed to look at how hypertension in a diabetic patient causes diabetic nephropathy.

In our previous study discussing the macrovascular complications of diabetes, we established that diabetes causes endothelial dysfunction, leading to thickening of blood vessels characterized by the narrowing of the lumen, as seen in arteriosclerosis. We also saw under the mechanism underlying microvascular complications that hypertension causes thickening and stiffening of the vessels, and the reason why the blood vessels thicken is so that they don't burst from the high pressure the blood exerts on them. As the capillaries (small blood vessels) narrow, the space through which blood passes in the arteries is reduced. When this thickening of the blood vessel and narrowing of the capillaries occur in the renal arteries, it will lead to low blood volume passing through the kidney.

As low blood volume passes through the nephron in the kidney, the kidney detects this low volume with the help of specific cells known as the ***juxtaglomerular cells***. As soon as these cells detect this low blood volume, the kidney then activates a special mechanism to increase blood pressure through the secretion of a special hormone known as renin, which will, in turn, increase blood volume to the kidney. It is important to remember that pressure is needed for effective filtration of blood in the kidney.

2. Mechanism of Renin Release

The RAAS system (Renin-Angiotensin-Aldosterone System) is a complex hormonal cascade that plays a key role in regulating blood pressure, fluid balance, and electrolyte levels in the body.

The mechanism of renin release is primarily triggered by decreased blood volume or low blood pressure, detected by specialized cells called juxtaglomerular cells located in the walls of the afferent arterioles of the nephron in the kidneys. When these cells sense reduced blood flow or pressure, they respond by releasing renin into the bloodstream.

Note

Renin is an enzyme produced by specialized cells in the kidneys called juxtaglomerular cells that is essential for regulating blood pressure and fluid balance in the body. Renin is released into the bloodstream in response to various stimuli, including low blood pressure, decreased blood volume, or low sodium levels.

Renin, in a cascade of events, will lead to the production of an enzyme called **Angiotensin II,** which is a potent *vasoconstrictor*, causing blood vessels to narrow. In this low–pressure state in the kidney, angiotensin II causes the efferent arteriole to constrict, retaining some pressure in the glomerulus of the kidneys. It equally stimulates the release of **aldosterone** from the adrenal glands. Aldosterone acts on the kidneys, promoting the reabsorption of sodium and water, thus increasing the body's overall blood volume and blood pressure.

Note

A vasoconstrictor is a substance or agent that causes blood vessels to narrow or constrict.

The overall effect of the RAAS (renin-angiotensin-aldosterone system) is to increase blood pressure and volume, ensuring adequate perfusion to vital organs, particularly the kidneys. This complex mechanism is crucial for maintaining homeostasis in response to changes in blood volume and pressure.

Over time, as the blood vessels continue to narrow due to hyperglycemia and hypertension and as blood pressure increases due to the RAAS system, the nephrons of the kidneys will start receiving larger and larger amounts of blood to filter, thereby causing an increase in glomerular filtration rate. Over time, this increased pressure will have some detrimental effects on the kidneys, some of which include:

Mesangial Expansion:
The prolonged increased flow of blood through the glomeruli

creates shear stress on the mesangial cells. Shear stress is the force exerted on the cells as a result of fluid flow. This mechanical stress triggers various cellular responses in the mesangial cells.

The shear stress activates signaling pathways within the mesangial cells. These pathways can lead to changes in gene expression and cellular behavior.

Note

Signaling pathways are intricate communication systems within cells that enable them to respond to various external stimuli or signals. These pathways involve a series of molecular events and interactions that transmit information from the cell's exterior to its interior, ultimately leading to specific cellular responses. Signaling pathways play a crucial role in regulating various biological processes, allowing cells to adapt and coordinate their activities in response to changes in their environment.

The activated mesangial cells release growth factors, which stimulate the fusion of the extracellular matrix proteins found in the mesangial cells. In response to signaling pathways and growth factors, mesangial cells start producing more extracellular matrix (ECM) proteins, whose primary function is to provide structural support to the glomerulus and is equally essential for maintaining its integrity.

It is important to remember that all these processes are occurring because the body is attempting to adapt to the high pressure in the kidney. This adaptation necessitates an increase in mesangial cells to withstand the elevated pressure.

The increased production of extracellular matrix (ECM) proteins results in mesangial expansion. This expansion involves the accumulation of matrix material in the mesangium, the region between the glomerular capillaries.

Mesangial expansion will alter the normal architecture of the glomerulus, leading to impaired filtration. This can result in reduced kidney function and may contribute to the progression of kidney diseases and the loss of the nephron.

Podocytopathy

Podocytopathy in the context of increased glomerular filtration rate (GFR) involves changes to the specialized cells called podocytes that line the glomerulus in the kidneys. Here's a simple yet detailed explanation of how podocytopathy occurs in the state of increased GFR:

Conditions such as glomerular hyperfiltration and hypertension can lead to an increase in blood flow through the glomerulus. The increased blood flow puts mechanical stress on the podocytes, which are crucial for maintaining the filtration barrier in the glomerulus.

In response to the increased blood flow, podocytes experience mechanical stretching and stress. Podocytes attempt to adapt to the increased demands by undergoing hypertrophy, which involves enlarging in size. Hypertrophy is a compensatory mechanism aimed at maintaining the integrity of the filtration barrier. Larger podocytes cover a greater surface area, attempting to compensate for the increased filtration demands.

Note

Hypertrophy refers to the enlargement or increase in size of an organ or tissue due to an increase in the size of its individual cells. This growth occurs in response to various stimuli, such as increased workload, hormonal stimulation, or exercise.

While podocyte hypertrophy initially serves a protective role, persistent stress and hypertrophy can lead to altered podocyte function. The podocytes may become dysfunctional over time, impairing their ability to regulate the filtration barrier effectively. Prolonged exposure to increased GFR and associated stressors can lead to podocyte damage, and this podocyte damage is called podocytopathy. Podocytopathy encompasses structural and functional changes in podocytes, some of which include podocyte loss, altered morphology, and a compromised ability to regulate the passage of substances through the filtration barrier.

Podocytopathy contributes to increased permeability of the filtration barrier, leading to the leakage of large molecules like proteins into the urine (**proteinuria**). The compromised filtration function and the presence of protein inside the urine are indicators of a dysfunctional kidney, and if left untreated, these changes can contribute to the progression of kidney diseases.

Glomerular Basement Membrane (GBM) thickening and sclerosis
In the state of increased glomerular filtration rate (GFR) caused by the RAAS system triggered by low blood pressure from arteries narrowed by hyperglycemia and hypertension, the glomerular basement membrane (GBM) undergoes structural changes that lead to thickening and sclerosis. When conditions such as glomerular hyperfiltration and hypertension elevate GFR, the heightened blood flow exerts mechanical stress on the GBM, triggering adaptive responses.

This stress activates signaling pathways within the glomerular cells, and in response, growth factors are released, stimulating the synthesis of extracellular matrix proteins. The accumulation of these matrix materials within the GBM results in its thickening, altering its normal structure.

Note:

Extracellular matrix proteins are a diverse group of molecules found outside of cells within tissues and organs in the body. These proteins form a complex network that provides structural support and organization to the surrounding cells. They play essential roles in maintaining tissue architecture, regulating cell behavior, and facilitating various cellular processes.

As the GBM thickens, it may become less permeable and less effective in its filtration function. Over time, persistent stress and structural changes can contribute to sclerosis, characterized by the progressive scarring and hardening of the glomerulus. The combination of GBM thickening and sclerosis compromises the integrity of the glomerular filtration barrier, leading to impaired kidney function.

Note

Sclerosis

In the context of increased glomerular filtration rate (GFR), sclerosis refers to a condition characterized by the progressive scarring and hardening of the glomerulus. It generally involves the gradual accumulation of scar tissue within the glomerulus, resulting in hardening and loss of normal function.

As these processes keep going on, it will lead to the loss of the nephron, which is the functional unit of the kidney. As more and more nephrons are destroyed, it will eventually lead to kidney failure.

The collective occurrence of mesangial expansion, podocytopathy, and glomerular basement membrane thickening will collectively cause irreversible loss of the nephron. As more and more nephrons are damaged due to hyperglycemia and hypertension, the kidney loses its ability to filter blood and

DIABETIC NEPHROPATHY

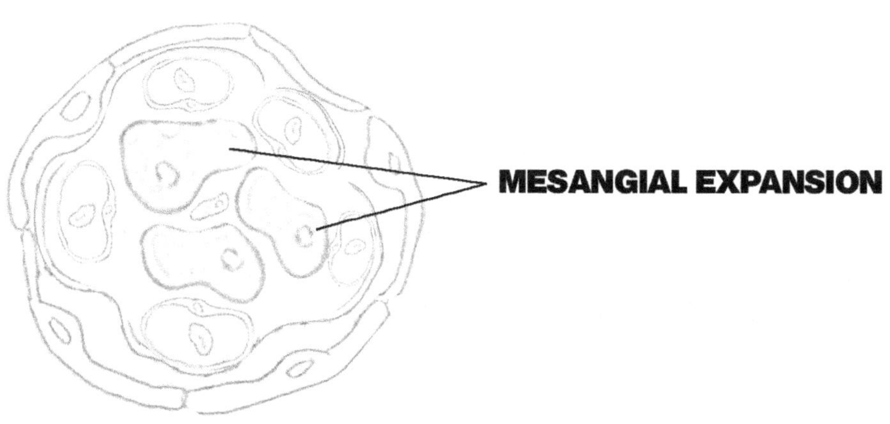

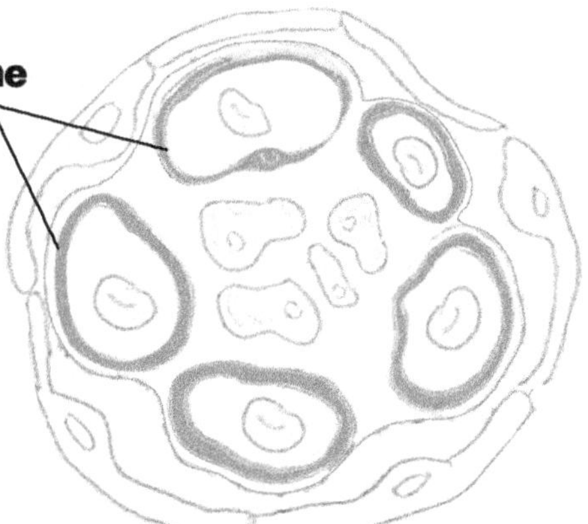

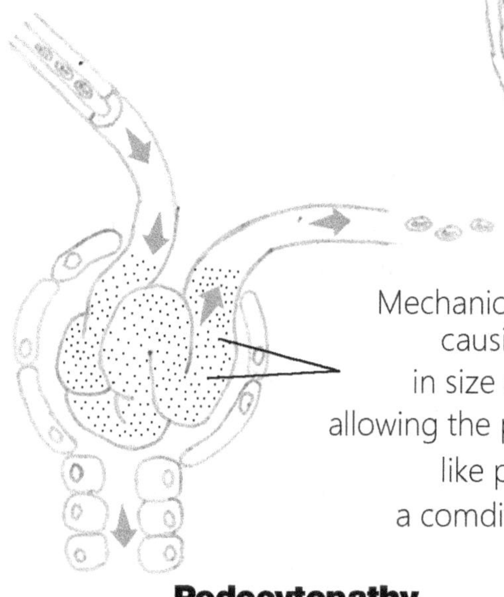

consequently loses its ability to regulate various other processes in the body. This is essentially what we call diabetic nephropathy.

Diabetic neuropathy

Diabetic neuropathy, as the name suggests, is nerve damage that occurs in people with diabetes. This affects almost everyone who has had diabetes for 15 to 20 years or more. Diabetes, especially when poorly managed over time, can lead to high levels of blood sugar (glucose), which can injure nerves throughout the body. In this section, we aim to look at diabetic neuropathy in depth and explain what makes it a very fatal disease.

One of the reasons why diabetic neuropathy is such a big subject is because, unlike the other complications of diabetes such as diabetic retinopathy and diabetic nephropathy, which often have clear-cut symptoms such as bleeding and leaky blood vessels in the eye (as seen in retinopathy) and larger molecules like protein that leak in the urine (microalbuminuria), as seen in nephropathy, their symptoms are very predictable.

Once detected, we know the progression and clinical manifestations, which makes it easy to control and manage. However, in the case of diabetic neuropathy that affects the nerves, it is not always easy to predict how it will express itself and which nerve it will affect. This is one of the many characteristics that make neuropathy so fatal.

Before we look at diabetic neuropathy in depth, let's have a small lesson on the nervous system of the body and how the nerves work, as it will help us to have a good grasp of diabetic neuropathy.

The Nervous System

The nervous system is a complex network of specialized cells, tissues, and organs that coordinate and control various functions in the body. It plays a crucial role in sensing stimuli from both the internal and external environment, processing information, and initiating appropriate responses.

The nervous system can be divided into two main parts: the central nervous system (CNS) and the peripheral nervous system (PNS).

The Central Nervous System:

The central nervous system (CNS) is a major division of the nervous system that consists of the brain and the spinal cord. It acts as the primary processing and control center for the whole nervous system. The CNS plays a crucial role in receiving, processing, and integrating information from various parts of the body. It is responsible for generating responses, coordinating movements, and regulating bodily functions. Essentially, the central nervous system is where sensory information is received, interpreted, and motor commands are initiated.

The Peripheral Nervous System

The peripheral nervous system (PNS) is a component of the nervous system that is situated outside the central nervous system (CNS). The peripheral nervous system consists of nerves and ganglia (clusters of nerve cell bodies) that extend throughout the body, connecting the CNS to various organs, tissues, and muscles. Its primary function is to facilitate communication between the central nervous system and the rest of the body.

The peripheral nervous system can be further divided into two main divisions: the sensory division (afferent) and the motor division (efferent).

The sensory division, also known as the afferent division, is a component of the peripheral nervous system that is responsible for transmitting sensory information from various parts of the body to the central nervous system (CNS). This division allows the nervous system to receive input from the environment and from within the body. Examples of sensory information include signals related to sight, smell, touch, and pain. Sensory neurons are the specific nerve cells within the sensory division that carry these signals to the CNS for processing.

Conversely, the motor division, also known as the efferent division, is another component of the peripheral nervous system that transmits signals from the central nervous system to muscles, glands, and other effector organs. This division enables the execution of voluntary and involuntary movements and responses. The motor division is further divided into the somatic nervous system and the autonomic nervous system.

Somatic Nervous System:
- The somatic nervous system is responsible for controlling voluntary movements and transmitting signals from the central nervous system (CNS) to skeletal muscles.
- It allows conscious control over skeletal muscles, enabling activities such as walking, talking, and moving the limbs.
- Sensory neurons within the somatic nervous system convey information about the external environment and the body's position to the CNS, contributing to our perception of touch, pain, and other sensations. Motor neurons in the somatic nervous system then carry signals from the CNS to skeletal muscles, triggering the desired voluntary movements.

Autonomic Nervous System:

- The autonomic nervous system (ANS) is responsible for regulating involuntary physiological processes and maintaining internal homeostasis.
- It controls various automatic functions such as heart rate, digestion, respiratory rate, and glandular activity.
- The autonomic nervous system is further divided into two main branches: the sympathetic division and the parasympathetic division.

The sympathetic division and the parasympathetic division are two branches of the autonomic nervous system (ANS), which is responsible for regulating involuntary physiological functions to maintain internal balance (homeostasis). These divisions often act in opposition to each other, and their activities are crucial for responding to various environmental and internal stimuli.

Sympathetic Division:

The sympathetic division is often associated with the "fight-or-flight" response, and prepares the body for an intensive physical activity. During activation of the sympathetic division:

- The heart's rate increases as it pumps more blood to the muscles.
- Pupils dilate to enhance vision.
- Airways dilate to increase oxygen intake.
- Blood flow is redirected to skeletal muscles, away from non-essential functions like digestion.
- The liver secretes glucose into the bloodstream for fast energy.

Overall, the sympathetic division prepares the body to deal with immediate challenges, whether physical or emotional.

Parasympathetic Division:
The parasympathetic division is often associated with the "rest and digest" response, promoting relaxation and recovery. During activation of the parasympathetic division:

- Heart rate decreases, promoting a state of rest.
- Pupils constrict to reduce their sensitivity to light.
- Airways constrict to slow down breathing.
- Blood flow is directed towards the digestive organs to enhance nutrient absorption and digestion.
- The body conserves energy and focuses on activities related to recovery and digestion.

The parasympathetic division counteracts the effects of the sympathetic division, promoting a return to a more relaxed state after a stressor has passed.

What is diabetic neuropathy?
Now, in the case of diabetic neuropathy, what happens is that hyperglycemia, through the processes of:

- Formation of Reactive Oxygen Species (ROS)
- Formation of Advanced Glycation End Products (AGEs)
- Endothelial Dysfunction
- Impaired Nitric Oxide (NO) Production
- Sorbitol and osmotic stress
- Release of Proinflammatory Cytokines
- Dyslipidemia
- Hyperglycemia–Induced Inflammation

will destroy the blood vessels supplying nutrients, oxygen, and other important components to the nerves of the body. This destruction can occur in any nerve around the body, but in most diabetic cases, we see that the destruction occurs in the peripheral nervous system (sensory nerves). When this destruction occurs, the nerve will be deprived of oxygen and nutrients, causing it to starve. As the nerve is deprived of nutrients over time, it will lead to damage to the nerve, causing it to be dysfunctional, and in most cases, it can lead to the death of the nerve.

Types of Diabetic Neuropathy

The main types of neuropathies we see in diabetes are:

Peripheral Neuropathy:

Peripheral neuropathy refers to a type of neuropathy that affects the peripheral nerves, which are the nerves outside the brain and spinal cord. Specifically, it often refers to damage or dysfunction of the sensory nerves, leading to a decrease or loss of sensation in the affected areas.

In the context of diabetes, peripheral neuropathy is a common complication where the sensory nerves in the extremities, particularly the feet, are affected. This can result in a gradual loss of sensation in the feet, making it difficult for individuals to detect injuries, pressure, or temperature changes in their feet.

When your feet are affected, you might start to lose feeling in them. Imagine stepping on a nail accidentally; usually, you'd pull your foot away quickly. But with neuropathy, especially in severe cases, an injury could lead to a diabetic foot ulcer. If this ulcer doesn't heal, it can turn into a serious foot infection, possibly causing gangrene and, in extreme situations, requiring amputation.

So, what starts as a simple decrease in foot sensation can end up leading to amputation. This highlights how important it is to understand neuropathy. Sometimes, instead of affecting feelings, it can impact the muscles or motor system. This can cause complications like foot drop, where the foot falls due to nerve and muscle issues. Other potential problems include a claw foot or a complete change in the foot's shape.

It's crucial to know that these issues usually happen in severe neuropathy cases. The good news is that, with proper diabetes management, you can often avoid these complications.

Cranial Neuropathy:

Cranial neuropathy refers to the dysfunction or damage to one or more of the cranial nerves, which are a set of twelve nerves that emerge directly from the brain. These nerves are responsible for controlling various functions in the head and neck regions, including those related to the eyes and facial muscles.

The eye has several muscles, each controlled by specific cranial nerves, including the third (oculomotor), fourth (trochlear), sixth (abducens), and seventh (facial) cranial nerves. When any of these nerves are affected, it can lead to various visual and facial abnormalities.

Examples of Cranial Neuropathy:

1. **Third Cranial Nerve (Oculomotor Nerve):**
   - If the third cranial nerve is affected, it can lead to a condition known as ptosis.
   - Ptosis involves the drooping or closing of one eyelid, resulting in a partially or completely closed eye.
2. **Facial Nerve (Seventh Cranial Nerve):**
   - Cranial neuropathy affecting the facial nerve can result in conditions such as Bell's palsy.
   - Bell's palsy is characterized by the paralysis or weakness of facial muscles on one side of the face, leading to the inability to move certain facial features.

Autonomic Neuropathy:

Autonomic neuropathy is a condition that affects the autonomic nervous system, which is responsible for controlling involuntary bodily functions such as heart rate, blood pressure, digestion, and sweating. This type of neuropathy occurs when there is damage to the nerves that regulate these automatic processes.

If you experience autonomic neuropathy, a sudden decrease in blood pressure upon standing may occur. This can lead to symptoms like dizziness and postural hypotension, creating a sensation of instability, often caused by autonomic neuropathy affecting the sympathetic system. Moreover, with autonomic neuropathy, you may not sweat enough in hot conditions. In these situations, some people may not sweat at all, which could be another sign of autonomic neuropathy.

In cases of severe autonomic neuropathy, individuals may not experience the typical symptoms associated with low blood sugar. Normally, when someone's blood sugar drops, they feel hungry, their heart palpitates, their fingers may tremble, and they start sweating. These signs prompt a person to eat, resolving the low-sugar situation. However, in severe autonomic neuropathy, the blood sugar can decrease from 5.55 mmol/L (100 mg/dL) to 2.22 mmol/L (40 mg/dL) without the person experiencing any symptoms. Suddenly, the blood sugar may plummet to 1.11 mmol/L (20 mg/dL), leading to fainting or a low sugar coma.

For individuals with severe autonomic neuropathy, proactive measures are necessary. Patients are advised to maintain their blood sugar levels at around 130–150 mg/dL (7.215–8.325 mmol/L) to prevent the risk of hypoglycemia. Fortunately, advancements in technology, such as small glucose monitoring patches, make this easier today. These patches, resembling caramel coins, can be attached to the hand to provide continuous glucose readings throughout the day and night, up to a hundred times per day.

Continuous glucose monitoring offers several advantages, including an ambulatory glucose profile. By examining the glucose trace, individuals can detect patterns and trends in their blood sugar levels. This is particularly beneficial during sleep, when potential blood sugar drops might go unnoticed. The information gleaned from the monitoring system allows individuals to adjust their medications, whether tablets or insulin, to prevent low blood sugar occurrences and avoid hypoglycemic comas.

Genital Neuropathy:
As its name suggests, this is a type of neuropathy that affects the genital area and occurs when the nerve responsible for erection is damaged. When genital neuropathy happens in men, they experience erectile dysfunction, while in women, they have reduced libido. If someone has uncontrolled diabetes for a long time, they will not have an erection at all. They therefore encounter difficulties with arousal or orgasm.

Diabetic neuropathy can also affect your bladder. Remember, it is a varied syndrome that can affect muscles and nerves all over the body. Typically, a person feels the urge to use the toilet when the bladder is half or three-fourths full. However, when the nerves controlling the bladder are affected, the sensation is diminished or completely absent. As a result, the bladder can fill up without the individual realizing it, leading to sudden urine release, a condition referred to as *incontinence.* In severe cases, the patient may remain unaware of the full bladder until the involuntary release of urine occurs.

Incontinence is a medical condition characterized by the inability to control the bladder or bowel movements. This might cause unintentional discharge of urine or feces. Incontinence can range from occasional leakage to a complete loss of bladder or bowel control. It can be caused by various factors such as muscle weakness, nerve damage, or underlying medical conditions.

Silent heart attacks

One scary thing about diabetic neuropathy is the fact that you can have a heart attack without even feeling the symptoms leading to the heart. Let's suppose the nerves in and around your heart have been affected. If you happen to have a heart attack, you will be completely unaware.

This is why, as a diabetes patient, it is very important to get regular checkups and always have your blood sugar levels in check so as to avoid and reduce the risk of getting the different neuropathic complications of diabetes we have seen so far.

These are some of the few neuropathies that can occur as a result of prolonged exposure to hyperglycemia.

Other Complications of Type 2 Diabetes

- **Hyperglycemic Hyperosmolar Non-Ketotic Syndrome (HHNS)**

While diabetic ketoacidosis is an acute complication of type 1 diabetes, hyperglycemic hyperosmolar non-ketotic syndrome (HHNS) is a very serious and acute complication of type 2, which has a mortality rate of 8–20%. In this section, we aim to discuss the clinical presentation and manifestation of HHNS and provide a detailed overview of the metabolic processes associated with this condition.

Note
A mortality rate of 8–20% means that out of every 100 individuals affected by a particular condition or disease, 8–20 of them will die as a result.

Just looking at the name Hyperglycemic Hyperosmolar Non-Ketotic Syndrome, we already have an idea of what this condition is and how it manifests. Nevertheless, the name alone doesn't portray some detailed key points associated with this condition.

Let's take a look at some key points to note when talking about HHNS.
When we talk about HHNS, the first point to note is that this condition is most common in type 2 diabetic individuals, and HHNS usually manifests itself sometime after the initial diagnosis of type 2 diabetes.

After an individual has been diagnosed with type 2 diabetes, they might start experiencing the symptoms of HHNS, some of which include fatigue, weight loss, extreme thirst, frequent urination, dehydration, hypotension, decreased turgor, confusion, or an altered mental status.

Now we ask ourselves, why is the patient experiencing these symptoms, and what is the underlying cause? In order to understand how HHNS causes the symptoms we listed above, we are going to dissect the name Hyperglycemic Hyperosmolar Non–Ketotic Syndrome (HHNS) and discuss the underlying metabolisms, and as we break down the name, we will see that one condition leads to another.

Hyperglycemic:
At this stage, it is no news that hyperglycemia (high blood glucose) is the defining characteristic of diabetes in both type 1 and type 2. We equally know that the reason for high blood glucose levels present in both type 1 and type 2 diabetes is due to the fact that in type 1 diabetes, insulin deficiency is absolute; there is no insulin produced, and this is due to a dysfunctional pancreas. Whereas in type 2 diabetes, insulin deficiency is relative, meaning that insulin is present in the bloodstream, but yet the cells of the body are resistant to its effects, and as such, glucose has a hard time entering the cells, causing hyperglycemia. Now that we have seen the first component responsible for the metabolism of HHNS, let's move on to the next.

Hyperosmolar:

One very important aspect to note about glucose is that it is an osmotically active element. This simply means that glucose has the ability to draw water to itself, and as such, where there is glucose in the body, you will find water. When an individual has high blood glucose, the glucose in the blood will tend to draw water from the surrounding cells, and this happens to keep the concentration of glucose in the blood constant.

When looking at the formation of sorbitol under the microvascular complications of type 2 diabetes, we mention that when glucose is in the cell, it draws water from the extracellular space so as to maintain the osmotic pressure of the cell, as this is necessary for the cell to function properly. But now, when this glucose is out of the cell and in the bloodstream due to insulin resistance, water will instead be pulled out of the cells to dilute the high concentration of glucose in the blood, and as this glucose travels around the body and into the kidney, it draws a large amount of water with it, which altogether will be expelled from the body as urine.

Normally, when blood is being filtered, the kidneys reabsorb all of the glucose back into the bloodstream, but in the case of severe hyperglycemia, the kidneys are not able to reabsorb all of the glucose, and so the excess glucose along with the water drawn from the cells and muscles will be spilled out as urine, and this explains why an individual suffering from diabetes urinates frequently.

As the body loses more and more water due to the excess glucose in the blood (hyperglycemia), the level of fluids in the body drops considerably, and this, in turn, increases the concentration of the solutes in the body. Some of these solutes

Some of these solutes include sodium, potassium, and even the glucose we have been talking about, causing more and more water to be pulled out of the cells of the body, worsening the dehydration. And this process in which the concentration of osmotically active solutes increases due to dehydration is known as hyperosmolarity, or high concentration of osmotically active solutes. And this explains why individuals suffering from diabetes experience intense thirst.

Non-Ketotic State:

If you have been following very closely, you will notice that there isn't much of a difference between Diabetic Ketoacidosis (DKA) and Hyperglycemic Hyperosmolar Non-Ketotic Syndrome (HHNS) at this stage, as they both exhibit metabolic features such as hyperosmolarity, hyperglycemia (absolute and relative insulin deficiency), dehydration, frequent urination, increased thirst, and electrolyte imbalance due to excessive fluid loss. The major differentiator between these two conditions is this non-ketotic state, which we will discuss shortly.

A very large majority of people with diabetes suffering from hyperosmolar hyperglycemic non-ketotic state (HHNS) are type 2 diabetes patients, and we know that in the early stages of type 2 diabetes, the pancreas is still functional and producing insulin. But now, one very important aspect to note in type 2 diabetes is that at the time of the diagnosis of type 2 diabetes, most people have half of their beta cell function gone due to the fact that their pancreas is overworking in an attempt to regulate the high blood glucose levels.

And as time goes by, you keep getting less and less beta cell function, which means that at some point, the level of insulin produced by the pancreas will be reduced considerably. Don't be confused; note that in type 2 diabetes, insulin is still being produced by the pancreas, but overtime, the output is relatively low compared to a healthy individual. This is the main difference between type 1 and type 2 diabetes and their acute complications (DKA and HHNS).

Throughout our studies on diabetes, we have seen that in type 1 diabetes, the cells of the body are in a state of starvation in the midst of plenty; there is enough glucose present in the bloodstream, but the cells of the body can't use this glucose for the production of energy. However, in type 2 diabetes, the cells are not starving but filled with glucose, and this causes them to exhibit a reduced response to the action of insulin to take up more glucose. Moreover, the pancreas function has been reduced so badly that the amount of insulin produced is relatively small and is still not able to shove all of the glucose in the bloodstream into the cells, all of which results in hyperglycemia.

As we have seen in Diabetic Ketoacidosis (DKA), when this hyperglycemia occurs in type 1 diabetes, the body will switch to an alternative source of energy and break down (metabolize) fat for energy. This process of fat breakdown will produce ketones, which are a byproduct of fat metabolism. Now these ketone bodies, also called ketoacids, result in metabolic acidosis. Hence the name diabetic ketoacidosis.

In type 2 diabetes, however, the insulin produced by the pancreas acts to inhibit the ketogenesis (formation of ketone bodies) pathway. The cells of the body in a type 2 diabetic patient are not starving, but, on the other hand, they are full of glucose, which has been accumulated through years of unhealthy eating habits and a sedentary lifestyle. And since the

In type 2 diabetes, however, the insulin produced by the pancreas acts to inhibit the ketogenesis (formation of ketone bodies) pathway. The cells of the body in a type 2 diabetic patient are not starving, but, on the other hand, they are full of glucose, which has been accumulated through years of unhealthy eating habits and a sedentary lifestyle. And since the cells are not in a state of starvation, there is no need for the body to switch to an alternative source of energy, as we see in type 1 diabetes. Hence the term hyperosmolar hyperglycemic non-ketotic state, since ketoacids are absent.

How to Treat Hyperosmolar Hyperglycemic Non-Ketotic State (HHNS)

Now that we know the metabolic processes, clinical presentation, and physiology (mechanism) of HHNS, let us use this knowledge to examine how HHNS can be treated. The first thing to note is that if someone is suffering from HHNS or is suspected to have HHNS, they should be rushed to the hospital and given intensive medical attention. The two major treatments for HHNS are:

IV Insulin (Intravenous Insulin)

Hyperosmolar hyperglycemic non-ketotic state (HHNS) is often associated with type 2 diabetes, and as such, patients suffering from HHNS have insulin resistance. Due to this insulin resistance, glucose is not being taken up in the cells, causing hyperglycemia, which is actually the main trigger for HHNS. The intravenous administration of insulin (insulin administered directly into the veins through injections) works to overcome this insulin resistance by forcing the cell filled with glucose to open up, thereby driving glucose out of the bloodstream and into the cells, reducing hyperglycemia. When the levels of glucose reduce, the levels of fluid loss caused by hyperglycemia will equally reduce, preventing hyperosmolarity from occurring.

IIV Rehydration (Intravenous Insulin)

Due to the severe fluid loss caused by hyperglycemia, it is important for bodily fluids to be restored so that certain metabolic processes occurring within the body can return to normal. In this case, aggressive IV rehydration (administration of fluid directly into the veins through injection) with fluids such as saline is important to alleviate the signs of low blood pressure and dehydration.

Slow Wound Healing in Diabetes

Slow healing of wounds is another complication commonly associated with prolonged exposure to hyperglycemia. One of the reasons why diabetic patients often experience slow wound healing is due to a lot of factors, but in this section, we aim to discuss a few:

- **Diabetic Neuropathy:**

Diabetic neuropathy is a condition where high levels of blood sugar damage the nerves, often affecting the extremities like the feet and hands. When we talk about the slow healing of wounds, diabetic neuropathy has an important role to play.

Nerve damage in diabetic nephropathy can lead to reduced or loss of sensation in the affected areas. This means that a person with diabetic neuropathy may not feel injuries or wounds as quickly as someone without this condition. Without prompt awareness, the body might not take immediate action to treat the wound, as it might not even know it's there due to nerve damage in the affected area due to diabetes.

- **Poor blood circulation:**

In a previous section of this chapter, we established that when you have diabetes, it narrows and destroys the blood vessels, which can cause poor blood circulation.

Poor blood circulation can slow down the wound healing process because blood plays a crucial role in the healing process. Here's a simple explanation:

When you get a wound, blood carries essential components like oxygen, nutrients, and immune cells to the injured area. Oxygen is crucial for cell function, nutrients provide energy for the healing process, and immune cells help fight off infections.

In the case of poor blood circulation due to narrowed blood vessels, the delivery of these essential elements to the wound site is compromised. When there's a shortage of oxygen and nutrients, cells involved in the healing process can't function optimally, and the immune response may be weakened.

Additionally, proper blood circulation helps remove waste products from the wound site. If circulation is impaired, waste products may accumulate, further hindering the healing process.

- **Gastroparesis**: This disorder affects the digestive system, causing delayed emptying of the stomach. High blood sugar levels can harm the neurons controlling the stomach muscles, leading to gastroparesis. Symptoms may include nausea, vomiting, bloating, and feeling full rapidly.
- **Sleep Apnea**: Individuals with diabetes are at a higher risk of developing obstructive sleep apnea, a condition characterized by pauses in breathing during sleep. Sleep apnea can further worsen blood sugar control and increase the risk of other complications, such as cardiovascular disease.
- **Depression and Anxiety:** Living with diabetes can be stressful due to the constant management of blood sugar

levels, medications, and potential complications. This stress, coupled with the physiological effects of diabetes on the brain, can increase the risk of depression and anxiety disorders.

- **Periodontal Disease**: Diabetes increases the risk of gum disease (periodontitis), characterized by inflammation and infection of the tissues surrounding the teeth. Poorly controlled diabetes impairs the body's ability to fight oral infections, leading to gum disease, tooth loss, and other dental complications.

- **Alzheimer's Disease and Dementia**: Emerging research suggests a link between diabetes and an increased risk of developing Alzheimer's disease and other forms of *dementia*. Chronic high blood sugar levels may contribute to the development of brain abnormalities and cognitive decline over time.

Note

Dementia is a generic term used to indicate a loss in mental ability severe enough to interfere with daily life. It is not a single disease but rather a combination of symptoms connected with a decrease in memory or other intellectual skills. These changes are often enough to reduce a person's ability to perform everyday activities. Dementia is caused by damage to brain cells, and the most common form is Alzheimer's disease.

- **Skin Conditions:** Diabetes can affect the skin in various ways, leading to conditions such as diabetic dermopathy (light brown patches on the skin), necrobiosis lipoidica diabeticorum (yellowish, waxy lesions on the skin), and fungal infections (such as candidiasis).

- **Gout**: Diabetes is associated with an increased risk of developing gout, a form of arthritis characterized by sudden and severe attacks of joint pain, swelling, and redness. High blood sugar levels promote the accumulation of uric acid crystals in the joints, triggering gout attacks

Note

Arthritis is a word used to describe a set of disorders that cause inflammation and pain in the joints. There are more than 100 different forms of arthritis, with osteoarthritis and rheumatoid arthritis being the most frequent.

Signs and Symptoms of Type 2 Diabetes

Throughout our exploration, we have witnessed the body's continuous efforts to maintain low and balanced levels of glucose in the bloodstream.

N. KEHSENI MARKBRON

CHAPTER THREE

Signs and Symptoms of Type 2 Diabetes

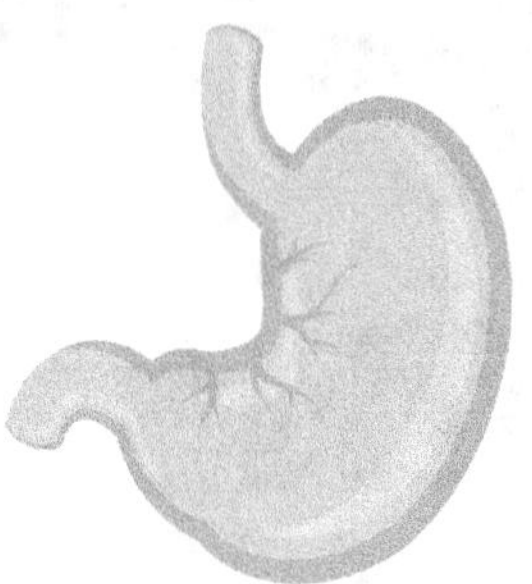

In this chapter, we aim to discuss the signs, symptoms, and clinical manifestations of type 1 and type 2 diabetes in depth. From subtle hints to more obvious signals, we'll walk through the different ways diabetes can show up and provide a detailed explanation of why they occur.

At this stage, it is certain that diabetes is characterized by hyperglycemia, which is high levels of glucose in the blood. As this chapter unfolds, we will come to understand that most of the signs and symptoms we see in the different stages of diabetes are mostly caused by these high levels of glucose.

Early Symptoms of Diabetes

Presence of glucose in urine (glucosuria)
So, from the past chapters, we've seen that during the body's attempt to manage excess glucose, insulin opens up the cells for glucose to go in and be converted to energy and commands the liver to store glucose as glycogen or convert this glucose into fats for more adequate storage. while glucagon prevents blood glucose levels from dropping too low by converting glycogen (stored glucose) back into glucose.

In a healthy individual, the normal fasting blood glucose

concentrations are between 3.9 mmol/L and 5.6 mmol/L (70–100 mg/dL), which just means that the blood glucose of a healthy individual must fall within this range after a period of fasting of at least 8 hours. Glucagon strives to keep the blood glucose above 3.9 mmol/L (70 mg/dL), and insulin always strives to keep the blood glucose below 5.6 mmol/L (100 mg/dL), although after eating foods rich in carbohydrates, it could rise to about 8 mmol/L (144 mg/dL), but only for a relatively short period of time.

Note: *Mmol/L means millimole per liter, and mg/dL means milligrams per deciliter.*

One very important aspect to note is that the renal threshold of glucose, i.e., the highest amount of glucose the nephron of the kidney can reabsorb in one liter of blood, is about 11 millimoles (198 mg/dL). This simply means that for every liter of blood that passes through your kidneys, the maximum amount of glucose the kidney can reabsorb back into the bloodstream is 11 millimoles. Now, this renal threshold does vary a bit between individuals; some might have a renal threshold of 10; others might be 12. But it's a fairly good rule of thumb that the renal threshold is around about 11 millimoles (198 mg/dL) of glucose per liter of blood.

This aspect is very important because once the glucose per liter of blood surpasses this renal threshold (11 mmol/L = 198 mg/dL), we start to see glucose present in urine, which is a serious call for concern and an indication of diabetes, as urine should **NOT** contain glucose at all in a normal and healthy individual.

In order to explain the renal threshold of glucose, let's briefly remind ourselves of how the nephron, which is the functional unit of the kidney, functions. From the physiology of the kidney, we saw that the nephron of the kidney has many functions, one of which is the filtration of blood. It is important to remember that per day, the kidneys filter about 180 liters of blood.

In a healthy kidney, when blood enters through the afferent arteriole, small molecules like water, glucose, creatine, protein, and electrolytes pass through the glomerulus into Bowman's capsule, and 99% of this filtrate produced from the glomerulus is reabsorbed back into the blood by the peritubular capillaries, with all of the glucose equally being reabsorbed.

Now, if your blood glucose level is 9 mmol/L (162 mg/dL), which basically means that for every liter of blood in your body, the quantity of glucose present is 9 millimoles, since it is lower than the renal threshold of glucose (11 mmol/L = 198 mg/dL), all of the 9 millimoles of glucose will be reabsorbed back into the blood, and no glucose will be found in the urine.

Let's suppose your blood glucose levels went up to 24 mmol/L of glucose. Again, this means that there's about 24 millimoles of glucose in the body per liter of blood. As your blood passes through the nephron and into the renal tubules, not all of the glucose will be reabsorbed into the blood, as 24 mmol/L is already way above the renal threshold, which stands at 11 mmol/L. Therefore, 11 mmol/L of blood glucose will be reabsorbed back into the bloodstream and 13 mmol/L of blood glucose will be passed out as urine, and this presence of glucose in urine is what we refer to as glucosuria, which is one of the very early symptoms of diabetes.

Frequent Urination (Polyuria):
Now, when the glucose in the blood exceeds the renal threshold of glucose, there will be a high-end concentration of glucose present in the renal tubules, ready to be passed out as urine.
One of the characteristics of glucose is that it is an osmotic molecule; it attracts water from the surrounding environment to itself through osmosis, and as it passes through the renal tubules,

it makes it very difficult for water to be reabsorbed back into the blood as more water is going to be retained to dilute the glucose in the renal tubules. This causes very large volumes of water to be passed out as urine, a condition known as diuresis. A diuresis is an abnormally large volume of urine being passed. This in turn causes frequent urination in the patient, a condition known as polyuria, which is one of the very early symptoms of diabetes.

Note

Osmosis: *Osmosis is the movement of solvent molecules (usually water) through a semipermeable membrane from a region of lower solute concentration to a region of higher solute concentration, thereby equalizing the concentrations on both sides of the membrane. In other words, it's the process by which water molecules move across a cell barrier to dilute the more concentrated solution.*

Another reason why a diabetic patient experiences frequent urination is due to insulin resistance. We know that when the cells of the body are resistant to the effects of insulin, glucose is not able to enter the cell, and as such, it accumulates in the bloodstream. We learned in chapter 2 under Hyperosmolar Hyperglycemic Non-Ketotic State (HHNS) that glucose has the ability to draw water to itself from the cells as it is a humectant. And as such, when glucose travels around the body, it draws a lot of water from the cells and muscles, and this water is eventually passed out as urine.

Excessive Thirst (Polydipsia):

The frequent urination, diuresis and the osmotic ability of glucose, which makes it hard for water to be reabsorbed from the kidney into the blood stream, will lead to a loss of fluids from the body, contributing to dehydration. In response, the body signals a heightened sense of thirst to encourage increased fluid intake. Excessive thirst, or polydipsia, is the body's way of trying to compensate for the fluid loss caused by increased urination, causing the individual to feel an intense and persistent need to drink large amounts of water.

Increased appetite (polyphagia)

Polyphagia, which refers to excessive hunger or increased appetite, is a symptom commonly associated with diabetes. However, it's important to note that not all individuals with diabetes experience polyphagia. The occurrence of polyphagia can depend on various factors, including the type of diabetes and the individual's specific circumstances.

In order to be able to understand how polyphagia occurs in diabetes, let's take a recap. Looking at Chapter 2 specifically, where we spoke about the overflow mechanism in an attempt to explain insulin resistance, we said that one of the main reasons why glucose can't get into the cell is due to the fact that the cells are packed with glucose, making it hard for more and more glucose to enter the already filled cells. This will thereby cause the cell to show some level of resistance to glucose since it is already full, and therefore more and more insulin will be needed to push in the excess glucose in the bloodstream into the cell.

While we had established that the underlying mechanism of type 1 diabetes is an autoimmune response, the immune system mistakenly attacks and destroys the beta cells in the pancreas, responsible for insulin secretion. This will result in very little or no Insulin, preventing glucose from entering the cells.

One very important factor to note here is that in type 1 diabetic patients, we see that the cells do not receive enough glucose because of the destruction of the beta cells in the pancreas responsible for producing insulin (absolute insulin deficiency). Whereas in type 2 diabetes, we notice that the reason why glucose can't get into the cell is due to the fact that there is so much glucose in the cell that has been accumulated over the years through unhealthy eating habits and a sedentary lifestyle (relative insulin deficiency). So, in one case, the cells are completely starving, and in the other, the cells are completely packed to capacity.

Now, whenever we look at type 1 and type 2 diabetic patients, we notice that polyphagia is more prominent in people suffering from type 1 diabetes than in type 2 diabetes, and this makes sense because, as we have seen above, the cells in type 1 diabetes are completely starved due to a complete lack of insulin. We have to remember that the cell uses glucose as fuel to produce energy through a complex series of processes, and as such, low or no glucose means little energy being produced.

As the brain starts sensing this low energy, it will then release hormones that will trigger hunger, pushing you to eat more and more, as the brain thinks that the reason for the lack of energy is a lack of nutrients within the body, whereas the real problem is that insulin is not being secreted to transport this glucose into the cell to produce energy. And this is the mechanism effectively responsible for causing increased hunger in type 1 diabetes patients.

One very good question to ask is: if the cells of type 2 diabetic patients are overfilled with glucose, then why do some of them experience polyphagia? Polyphagia can also be a symptom of type 2 diabetes, but it might not be as prominent as in type 1 diabetes.

Various research and statistics show that about 90% of type 2 diabetic patients are affected by a degree of obesity, and this finding explains why polyphagia may occur in some type 2 diabetic patients.

There are two hormones in the body responsible for hunger and satiety: ghrelin and leptin, respectively. Now, when an individual with type 2 diabetes suffers from obesity, there are two major dysregulations in the body that can alter their hunger and satiety hormones. These two conditions are insulin resistance and leptin resistance. Note here that leptin is responsible for the feeling of satiety after a meal.

Leptin is a hormone secreted by fat cells; it is secreted after you have eaten a meal and gives the brain the feeling of satiety, causing you to feel full after a meal. Leptin resistance is a very common condition seen in obese people. If your body doesn't respond to leptin effectively (leptin resistance), your ability to feel full after a meal becomes altered, leading to a sensation of continuous hunger even after a meal.

When someone who is diabetic has both insulin and leptin resistance combined, it seriously messes up their body's ability to regulate hunger and satiety. We will not really expound on how leptin resistance comes about in this chapter, but it is rather necessary to understand that polyphagia in type 2 diabetes is primarily caused by an impairment in the hormone leptin, responsible for feeling satisfied after a meal.

Common Symptoms of Diabetes

Unexplained Weight Loss
Now, stemming from the little recap we had above on why glucose doesn't get into the cells of both type 1 and type 2

diabetes patients, it makes complete sense for a type 1 diabetic patient to have unexplained weight loss. This is due to the obvious reason that the cells in a type 1 diabetic patient are completely starving due to the fact that there is an absence of insulin to transport glucose into the cell. As this insulin deficiency continues, the body will turn to fats and proteins in the muscle cells and adipose tissues for energy, which causes the muscle to shrink considerably and fat cells in the adipose tissues to be used up, causing the patient to experience severe weight loss.

Another factor contributing to more weight loss is the fact that as your body breaks down these fats, it also breaks down glycogen (a compact form of glucose suitable for storage) into glucose. One thing to remember about glucose is its ability to retain water. So, as glycogen is broken down into glucose, a lot of water will be drawn out of your muscle cells, causing them to shrink even more. So a combination of fat breakdown for energy and the loss of water from the cells as glucose travels through the blood will lead to weight loss. In type 1 diabetic patients.

Now let's try to figure out why, even though unexplained weight loss is more frequent in type 1 diabetes, some type 2 diabetic patients experience this condition.

At the time of the diagnosis of type 2 diabetes, most people have half of their beta cell function gone due to the fact that their pancreas is overworking in an attempt to regulate their high blood glucose levels. With proper diet and exercise, your beta function can return to normal, but most newly diagnosed individuals often don't respect the necessary activities required to increase their beta function.

And as time goes by, you keep getting less and less beta cell function, which means that at some point, you will not have enough insulin to transport glucose to the cells in order to produce energy. When this happens, glucose will build up in the blood (hyperglycemia), and this glucose being an osmotically active molecule will pull water from the muscles and cells of the body, as we have seen in hyperglycemic hyperosmolar non-ketotic syndrome (HHNS), causing them to shrink considerably and hence causing the individual to lose a lot of weight and muscle mass even though the cells are packed with glucose.

Fatigue

Fatigue can be a symptom of diabetes due to several interconnected reasons. The relationship between diabetes and fatigue can be explained by various factors:

- **Poor Sleep Quality:** Diabetes can be associated with sleep disturbances. The need for frequent urination during the night due to elevated blood sugar levels can disrupt sleep, leading to fatigue.
- **Narrowed blood vessels:** One very similar complication in diabetes is the fact that when an individual has diabetes, they tend to have inflammation in their blood vessels. A condition caused by atherosclerosis leading to the narrowing of the blood vessels. We know that blood is responsible for supplying the cells of the body with different nutrients, hormones, and oxygen, and oxygen is a key element in the conversion of glucose to energy. As blood vessels are narrowed, the volume of blood supplied to some organs and cells of the body is reduced, and with reduced blood supply, there is reduced oxygen and nutrient supply, all of which will lead to reduced energy production, resulting in fatigue.
- **Insulin Deficiency:** In type 1 diabetes, the pancreas can't

produce enough insulin, resulting in high blood glucose and a reduced ability of the cells to utilize glucose for energy. As a result, there will be a decrease in the energy output, resulting in fatigue.

There are many more factors contributing to fatigue in diabetes, but we will limit ourselves to these few.

Blurred vision

One of the very early signs of diabetes is blurred vision. Let's look at three ways in which high blood glucose can cause blurred vision in individuals suffering from diabetes.

- **Sorbitol**

When you have high blood glucose in your bloodstream, it constantly floats around the fluid in your eye (aqueous humor). The lens of the eye, responsible for focusing light onto the retina, will absorb this glucose. If you can recall one of the properties we discussed about cells, it is that they have the ability to transform glucose into a sugar alcohol molecule known as sorbitol through a special enzyme. One thing about sorbitol is that it is an osmotically active molecule (osmolyte), meaning it draws water from the surrounding fluids outside the cell and can change the osmotic pressure of the cell through osmotic stress.

Now, the conversion of glucose to sorbitol is a normal cellular process happening within the cell, and usually, it doesn't have a major consequence in a normal and healthy individual. In a diabetic patient, however, as more and more glucose is converted to sorbitol in the lens of the eye, It can result in an abnormally significant alteration in osmotic pressure, leading to cellular swelling.

When this osmotic pressure builds up in the lens, it causes the lens to change shape and get thicker. Now, luckily, this can be temporary and reversible, especially when you get your blood sugar under control. This will get rid of that excess fluid that got sucked into the cells of the lens and get rid of the sorbitol. Causing the lens to return to its regular shape.

- **Cataracts**

Having diabetes can potentially increase the risk of developing a cataract. A cataract is a medical condition characterized by the clouding of the natural lens in the eye, which leads to a gradual loss of vision. The lens, located behind the iris and pupil, is responsible for focusing light onto the retina at the back of the eye, allowing us to see clearly. Cataracts develop when the proteins in the lens of the eye begin to clump together, causing the lens to become cloudy. This cloudiness interferes with the normal passage of light, resulting in blurred or hazy vision.

When someone has diabetes for a long time, the excess level of glucose found in the eye will react with the red blood cells and the protein in the lens of the eye in a process called glycation. This reaction between glucose, hemoglobin, and protein will undergo a chain of reactions, modifications, and arrangements to form a more complex and stable molecule known as AGEs (Advanced Glycation End Products).

One thing about AGEs is that they are very sticky compounds, and due to this, they tend to form clogs as they circulate around the eye, especially in the tiny blood vessels of the eye. This advanced glycation end product (AGE) also causes the proteins in the lens of the eye to clump together, causing the lens to become cloudy and resulting in a cataract. It is very important to note that cataracts aren't reversible, and when they get to a stage of visual loss, surgery is usually performed to clear up the cataract.

Some other causes of cataracts include old age, prolonged exposure of the eye to UV radiation, some genetic conditions, and eye injuries.

- **Diabetic Macula Edema (DME)**

The macula is a small, highly sensitive area at the center of the retina in the eye. It is responsible for central vision, allowing us to see fine details clearly. The macula is essential for activities such as reading, recognizing faces, and seeing objects directly in front of us.

Diabetic macular edema (DME), in simple terms, involves the swelling and fluid buildup in the macula. It often occurs due to the damage to the blood vessels in the eye caused by processes such as increased vascular permeability and inflammation, all of which can lead to leakage from the blood vessels in the eye. When fluid accumulates in the macula due to diabetes-related changes in the blood vessels of the eye, it can cause the macula to swell. This swelling can lead to blurred or distorted central vision, making it difficult to see fine details. Diabetic macular edema is a potential complication of diabetic retinopathy, and so regular eye check-ups are important for the early detection and management of DME to help preserve vision.

Other symptoms of diabetes include:
- **Frequent infections:** Diabetes can weaken the immune system, making individuals more susceptible to infections, particularly in the skin, gums, or urinary tract.
- **Tingling or numbness in extremities:** Diabetes can cause nerve damage (neuropathy), leading to sensations of tingling, numbness, or pain, especially in the hands and feet.
- **Itchy skin:** Dry skin and itching, particularly around the genital area, can be a symptom of diabetes.

- **Recurrent yeast infections:** Women with diabetes may experience more frequent yeast infections, as elevated blood sugar levels create an environment conducive to fungal growth.
- **Digestive problems:** Diabetes can affect the nerves in the digestive system, leading to issues such as constipation or diarrhea.
- **Irritability:** Fluctuations in blood sugar levels can affect mood and energy levels, leading to irritability or mood swings.
- **Poor concentration and memory:** Some people with diabetes may experience difficulties in concentration and memory due to changes in blood sugar levels that affect the brain.

Diagnosing And Testing of Type 2 Diabetes

N. KEHSENI
MARKBRON

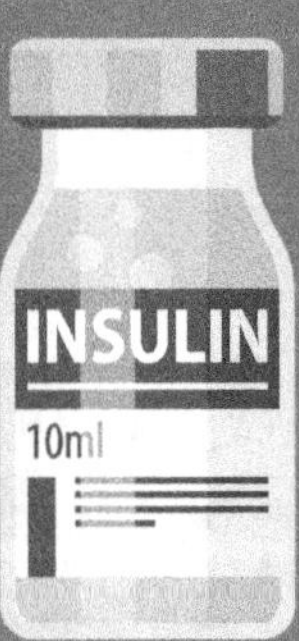

Before someone is diagnosed with diabetes, they usually present with one of the following states:

Diagnosing And Testing of Type 2 Diabetes

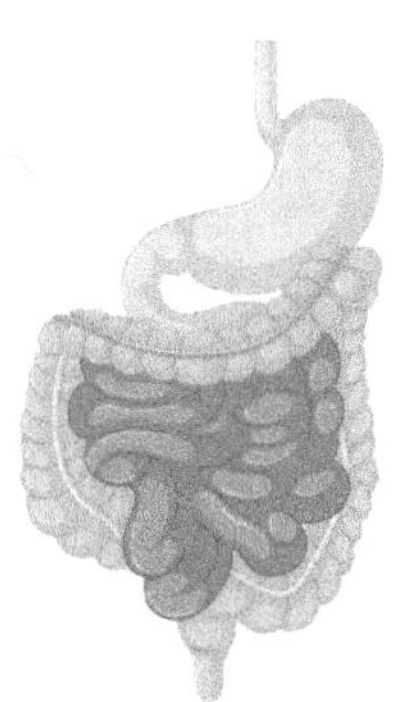

In the previous chapter, we discussed the signs and symptoms of diabetes, exploring all the common indicators that accompany the condition. When an individual starts experiencing the signs and symptoms we discussed in the previous chapter, it is important to get their blood glucose checked, as these signs are a major indication that the individual might be suffering from diabetes. It is important to note that irrespective of the type of diabetes an individual might have, they are all diagnosed in the same way.

In this chapter, we aim to look at all the necessary diagnoses and tests important to detecting and controlling diabetes. We equally aim to explain all the necessary criteria for pronouncing someone as diabetic or prediabetic.

Before someone is diagnosed with diabetes, they usually present with one of the following states:

1. Acute State:

This state of diabetes is very severe, causing the patient to become sick for a relatively short period of time. Symptoms at this stage include vomiting, nausea, and abdominal pain. This acute state is characterized by complications like diabetic ketoacidosis (DKA), as seen in type 1 diabetes, and hyperglycemic hyperosmolar non-ketotic state (HHNS), as seen in type 2 diabetes.

2. Subacute State:

The subacute stage is usually characterized by a mild feeling of unwellness over a period of weeks or months. Some symptoms that can accompany this feeling of unwellness may include fatigue, increased thirst, frequent urination, and weight loss. This subacute state is the most common form of presentation leading to the diagnosis of type 1 diabetes, and it accounts for about 70% of diagnoses in type 1. This state is also present in type 2 diabetes, but patients may not experience weight loss as much.

3.Asymptomatic state:

An asymptomatic state is a state in which an individual could be diabetic, yet they don't present any diabetes-related symptoms. Therefore, diabetes is usually diagnosed using an asymptomatic screening test. An asymptomatic screening test is a medical examination or diagnostic test performed on individuals who do not show any symptoms of a particular condition or disease. The purpose of these screenings is to detect potential health issues early, even before symptoms become apparent.

In the context of diabetes, asymptomatic screening tests might involve measuring blood glucose levels in individuals who do not exhibit signs of diabetes, aiming to identify any abnormal blood sugar levels that could indicate the early stages of the condition. These screenings are valuable for preventive healthcare, helping to catch and address health concerns in their early and potentially more manageable stages.

Type 2 diabetes affects nearly 10% of the world's population, and due to its frequent occurrence and severe complications, individuals who are more susceptible to having the disease, especially those with its associated risk factors, should undergo regular checkups. Asymptomatic screening tests are the most common way in which type 2 diabetes is diagnosed.

Diagnostic Criteria

Irrespective of the type of diabetes you have and the different complications associated with it, a lab test is necessary for the diagnosis of diabetes. Several types of laboratory tests exist for the diagnosis of diabetes, but we are going to look at these two types in depth.

Types of Diabetes Test

1. Blood Glucose Levels:

When someone has diabetes, his or her blood glucose is abnormally high, and this hyperglycemia accounts for 95% of the complications and symptoms a diabetic patient experiences.

So, one of the main indicators of diabetes is high blood glucose, and this is one of the components tested in the blood when someone is suspected of having diabetes.

There are several tests that measure blood glucose, and the results are not always the same for all the tests. Below are some major tests used to measure blood glucose

The Fasting Blood Sugar Test (FBS): The Fasting Blood Sugar Test (FBS) is a simple yet crucial test to measure glucose levels in the blood after an overnight fast. Here's a step-by-step explanation:

Preparation:

- **Fasting Period:** You are required to fast for at least 8 hours before the test. This usually means no food or drink, except water, during this period. It's commonly done overnight, and the test is often scheduled for the morning.

Procedure:

- **Visit to the Lab or Healthcare Provider:** Schedule an appointment with your healthcare provider or a lab for the test. Inform them of any medications you are currently taking, as certain medications can affect blood glucose levels.

- **Blood Sample Collection:** Upon arrival, a healthcare professional will collect a blood sample. They will typically use a needle to draw blood from a vein, which is often in the arm

- **Analysis:**The blood sample is subsequently sent to a laboratory for analysis. In the lab, the blood is tested to measure the concentration of glucose.

- **Interpretation of Results:** The results will be provided in milligrams of glucose per deciliter of blood (mg/dL) or millimoles per liter (mmol/L), depending on the unit of measurement used in your region.

Normal Range:

- Normal fasting blood sugar levels typically fall in the range of 70 to 99 mg/dL (3.9 to 5.5 mmol/L). However, these values can vary slightly between different labs.

Post-Test:

Consultation:

- Your healthcare provider will discuss the results with you and interpret them in light of your overall health.
- Elevated levels may indicate prediabetes or diabetes, while lower levels may be a sign of hypoglycemia.

Next Steps:

- Based on the results, your healthcare provider may recommend further tests, lifestyle changes, or medication if necessary.

The Random Blood Sugar Test: The Random Blood Sugar Test is a quick and convenient way to check your blood glucose levels at any time of the day, regardless of when you last ate. Here's a step-by-step explanation:

Procedure:

Visit to the Lab or Healthcare Provider:

- Schedule an appointment with your healthcare provider or a lab for the test.
- This test does not require fasting, so you can have it done at any time during the day.

Blood Sample Collection:

- Upon arrival, a healthcare professional will collect a blood sample. They will typically use a needle to draw blood from a vein, which is often in the arm.
- Unlike fasting tests, you don't need to have abstained from food or drink for this one.

Analysis:

- The blood sample is thereafter sent to a laboratory for analysis.
- In the lab, the blood is tested to measure the concentration of glucose.

Interpretation of Results:

- The results will be provided in milligrams of glucose per deciliter of blood (mg/dL) or millimoles per liter (mmol/L), depending on the unit of measurement used in your region.

Normal Range:

- Normal random blood sugar levels can vary, but they are typically below 200 mg/dL (11.1 mmol/L). However, these values can vary slightly between different labs.

Post-Test:

Consultation:

- Your healthcare provider will discuss the results with you and interpret them in light of your overall health.
- Elevated levels may indicate prediabetes or diabetes, while lower levels may be a sign of hypoglycemia.

Next Steps:

- Based on the results, your healthcare provider may recommend further tests, lifestyle changes, or medication if necessary.

Oral Glucose Tolerance Test (OGTT): The two-hour glucose tolerance test, also known as Oral Glucose Tolerance Test (OGTT), is performed to evaluate how well your body processes glucose. It involves drinking a sugary solution, and blood samples are taken at intervals to measure the rise and fall of glucose levels. Here's a detailed explanation:

Preparation:

- **Fasting Period:**
- You'll be instructed to fast for at least 8 hours before the test. It's commonly done overnight, and the test is usually scheduled for the morning.

Avoiding Certain Substances:

- You may be asked to avoid certain medications, caffeine, and strenuous exercise for a day or two before the test, as they can affect glucose levels.

Procedure:

Baseline Blood Sample:

- When you arrive at the healthcare facility, a baseline blood sample is taken to measure your fasting blood glucose level.

Drinking the Glucose Solution:

- After the initial blood sample, you'll be given a glucose solution to drink. The solution contains a predetermined amount of glucose (usually 75 grams).
- The taste can be sweet, so be prepared for that.

Waiting Period:

- You'll then wait for about 2 hours. It's essential to stay at the testing facility during this time, and you should avoid eating or drinking anything except water.

Additional Blood Samples:

- Blood samples will be taken at specific intervals, typically every 30 minutes or hourly, for the next 2 hours.
- These samples help monitor how your body processes the glucose from the solution.

Analysis:

- The blood sample is thereafter sent to a laboratory for analysis.
- The glucose levels in each sample are measured to assess how your body metabolizes glucose over time.

Post-Test:

Consultation:

- Following the test, your healthcare professional will review the results with you.
- Elevated glucose levels at certain time points may indicate impaired glucose tolerance or diabetes.

Next Steps:

- Depending on the results, your healthcare provider may recommend further tests, lifestyle changes, or medication if necessary.

Note:

It is important to note that a random blood sugar test cannot be used to diagnose pre-diabetes. You need either a fasting blood glucose test or an oral glucose tolerance test.

A blood glucose level greater than or equal to 200 mg/dL (11.1 mmol/L) is indicative of diabetes.

2. Hemoglobin A1c (HbA1c) Test:

One major process that occurs when you have high levels of glucose sitting in your bloodstream for very long periods of time is glycation. Glycation is the non-enzymatic attachment of glucose to certain surrounding molecules, especially proteins. Glucose is a reactive molecule and therefore tends to bind itself with surrounding proteins and even fats. One very interesting thing about this reaction of glucose and protein molecules is that no enzyme is required for the binding to take place, and this is what we mean by a non-enzymatic reaction. One major protein that binds to glucose during the glycation process is hemoglobin. Hemoglobin is the protein found within the red blood cells, and it is responsible for the red color we see in blood. This is so because hemoglobin contains a pigment made of iron and heme, giving it its red color.

This attachment of glucose to hemoglobin forms what's called glycated hemoglobin, or hemoglobin A1c (HbA1c). You can think of glycated hemoglobin as a coating formed by glucose found on the surface of a red blood cell. Now, this process occurs slowly, more like rust on iron. Let's say you keep a metal spoon outside for a while; after some time, you will notice that rust has started forming on the spoon, and the longer the spoon stays outside and is exposed to moisture, the more rust will be formed on it. And this is exactly what happens with glycation.

While glycated products (glycated hemoglobin) have a lot of negative impacts on the body, their discovery has revolutionized the way we understand diabetes and has helped us to be able to study and control diabetes more effectively. This is so because of the invention of the HbA1c test. The HbA1c test was invented around 1979 or 1980. Before then, only the different blood sugar tests we mentioned above were performed to diagnose diabetes. And while this was convenient at the time, it didn't provide much insight into how well the patient was managing his diabetes.

An HbA1c test, also known as a hemoglobin A1c or glycated hemoglobin test, is a blood test used to measure the average blood sugar levels over the past 2 to 3 months. In other words, this test gives the healthcare provider or doctor an insight into how well this patient is managing his or her blood glucose over the span of 2–3 months. The HbA1c test specifically measures the percentage of hemoglobin cells (red blood cells) that have glucose attached to them.

Now remember, the formation of glycated hemoglobin occurs when glucose sits in the blood for a long time, and glycation is a slow process. And so, the longer glucose sits in the blood, the more red blood cells will be glycated, while if your blood glucose is well controlled, you won't experience glycation of red blood cells as much. And this test essentially shows you how well you have controlled your blood glucose over the last 2–3 months.

Normal HbA1c levels are typically below 5.6%. In a prediabetic individual, the HbA1c level usually ranges between 5.7 and 6.4%. And an HbA1c level of 6.5% and above is consistent with diabetes. It is always advised to keep the HbA1c level below 7%. If an individual has an HbA1c level between 10% and 12%, this is a clear indication that his blood glucose has never been controlled over the last 2–3 months. I mentioned earlier that the HbA1c test has greatly revolutionized the way we understand and manage diabetes. So now let's look at why this test is such a breakthrough in the field of diabetes.

Over the years, a lot of studies have been conducted to find the relationship between HbA1c levels and the different complications associated with diabetes. Many of these studies confirm that as your HbA1c levels go above 7%, your risk of developing diabetic complications (retinopathy, neuropathy, nephropathy, slow healing of wounds, cardiovascular diseases, etc.) increases.In fact, for every one percent increase in your HbA1c levels, such as from 7 to 8, from 8 to 9, and so on, your risk of developing the different complications associated with diabetes increases by 25–30%.

So, suppose your HbA1c levels go up to 11–12%, you're almost at a 100% risk of developing the different complications associated with diabetes, and this is why HbA1c tests are repeated every three months to ensure that your blood glucose levels are under control. These different studies also suggest that if you can manage to keep your HbA1c levels under 7%, you will never develop the risks associated with diabetes. And this is why HbA1c tests are so important.

How is diabetes diagnosed?
The presentation and results of a blood glucose test are very important in the diagnosis of diabetes, but they are not enough to declare someone diabetic. There are two ways in which someone with diabetes can be diagnosed.

1. If an individual experiences the states of diabetes, whether acute or subacute, then only one positive diabetes test, either the blood sugar test or the HbA1c test, is necessary to diagnose them with diabetes.
2. If the individual is asymptomatic, then two positive diabetes tests separated by one week are necessary for the diagnosis of diabetes.

Glucometers

Throughout our studies on diabetes, we have seen that having high levels of blood glucose can be very fatal for diabetic patients, and this is the reason why it is important not only to constantly monitor your blood glucose but also to always keep them at a safe and manageable range. Usually, blood glucose tests are mostly carried out in the hospital, but for type 1 diabetes patients, whose diabetes is a result of the destruction of the beta cells in the pancreas responsible for the production of insulin and not a sedentary lifestyle, their blood glucose levels are hardly ever constant. As such, it can fluctuate between hyperglycemia (high blood glucose) and hypoglycemia (low blood glucose) without them ever noticing, and this is one reason why diabetes patients, especially type 1 diabetes patients, are supposed to constantly have an idea of their blood glucose level so as to know how to stabilize it.

The problem of unstable blood sugar levels has led to the invention of some special devices necessary for testing and monitoring blood sugar levels. These devices are called glucose meters, or glucometers. A glucometer is a medical device that typically measures the concentration of glucose in the blood. A sample of blood is placed on a disposable test strip that is inserted in the glucometer, where a chemical reaction of glucose alters the electrical conductivity of the test strip, which in turn allows the device to determine the concentration of glucose in the blood.

History of Glucometers

Glucometers, devices used to measure blood glucose levels, have a rich history of development dating back to the mid-1800s. Initially, attempts to quantify glucose in urine set the stage for modern diabetes care. In 1908, Benedict's introduction of a copper reagent for urine glucose marked a significant milestone in commercializing urine glucose testing. This method, though cumbersome, persisted for over 50 years with modifications.

The landscape changed in 1945 with the advent of Clinitest, which simplified the process with a modified copper reagent tablet. This advancement allowed for easier glucose oxidation and semi-quantitative assessment of glycosuria through color changes in the heated solution.

A pivotal moment arrived in 1965 when Ames introduced the Dextrostix, the first blood glucose test strip utilizing glucose oxidase. Although initially for physician use, this innovation laid the groundwork for home glucose monitoring. By 1980, the Dextrometer was launched, featuring a digital display and catering to home use, marking a shift towards patient-centered glucose monitoring.

Throughout the 1980s and beyond, advancements in glucometer

technology continued. These included improvements in precision, accuracy, and user-friendliness, with meters and strips requiring less blood becoming widely available and affordable. This period also saw the rise of self-monitoring of blood glucose (SMBG) as a standard of care, particularly for type 1 diabetes patients.

Continuous Glucose Monitoring

As time went on, scientists understood that the fingerstick glucose reading was not very convenient to monitor blood glucose, as it only provided the blood glucose reading for a particular point in time and didn't really tell a whole lot about the trend in the blood glucose levels of diabetic patients. The evolution of home glucose monitoring took a leap with the introduction of continuous glucose monitoring (CGM) in 1999. A CGM system, or Continuous Glucose Monitoring System, is a device used to continuously monitor and track glucose levels in the body. Initially,

CGM devices required calibration with fingerstick measurements (to prick the skin and obtain drops of blood for testing). However, innovations such as the Glucowatch Biographer and subsequent real-time CGM systems by Medtronic and Dexcom (companies focusing on diabetes management) pushed the boundaries of glucose monitoring technology.

By 2012, Dexcom's G4 Platinum (a type of continuous glucose monitoring system) introduced improved accuracy, paving the way for future advancements like the G5 Mobile and G6. Medtronic also made strides with integrated pump-sensor systems, culminating in the development of hybrid closed-loop devices. Abbott's FreeStyle Libre Pro (a continuous glucose monitoring (CGM) system consisting of a handheld reader and a glucose sensor worn on your arm), introduced in 2016, marked a significant milestone by eliminating the need for fingerstick testing during wear, setting a new standard in professional CGM systems.

In less than two decades, CGM has revolutionized diabetes management, especially for type 1 diabetes. The vast and unequivocal evidence supporting CGM underscores its critical role in modern diabetes care.

How do CGMs work?

Continuous glucose monitors (CGMs) typically consist of a handheld reader and a glucose sensor worn on your arm. They work by inserting a tiny sensor under the skin, usually on the abdomen or arm. This sensor measures glucose levels in the interstitial fluid (the fluid surrounding the body's cells) rather than directly in the blood. When there is sugar in the bloodstream, it moves from the blood vessel into the interstitial fluid beneath the skin, where it is detected by this tiny sensor. The sensor then sends this data to the transmitter worn on the body, which wirelessly communicates with a receiver or a smartphone app. Users can see their glucose levels in real-time and track changes over time. With CGM, people living with diabetes always know what their blood sugar is. Some CGMs also provide alerts for high or low glucose levels, helping users manage their diabetes more effectively.

Other types of diabetes tests

1. **Lipid profile**: Measures levels of cholesterol and triglycerides in the blood, which are important for assessing cardiovascular health.
2. **Kidney function tests:** Such as serum creatinine, blood urea nitrogen (BUN), and urine albumin-to-creatinine ratio (ACR), are used to assess kidney function and screen for diabetic

nephropathy.

1. **Liver function tests:** Such as alanine transaminase (ALT), aspartate transaminase (AST), and alkaline phosphatase (ALP), are used to assess liver health, as diabetes can affect liver function.
2. **Urine microalbumin test:** To detect small amounts of protein (albumin) in the urine, which can be an early sign of kidney damage in diabetes.
3. **Comprehensive metabolic panel (CMP):** Includes tests for electrolytes, kidney function, liver function, and glucose levels, providing a broad overview of metabolic health.
4. **Thyroid function tests:** Such as thyroid-stimulating hormone (TSH), free thyroxine (T4), and triiodothyronine (T3) to assess thyroid function, as thyroid disorders are more common in people with diabetes.
5. **Eye examination:** Including a dilated eye exam and retinal photography to screen for diabetic retinopathy, a complication affecting the eyes.
6. **Peripheral neuropathy assessment:** Such as nerve conduction studies or monofilament testing to assess nerve function, as diabetes can lead to peripheral neuropathy.
7. **Foot examination:** To check for signs of neuropathy, peripheral arterial disease, and foot ulcers, which are common complications of diabetes.

Medicines & Treatment

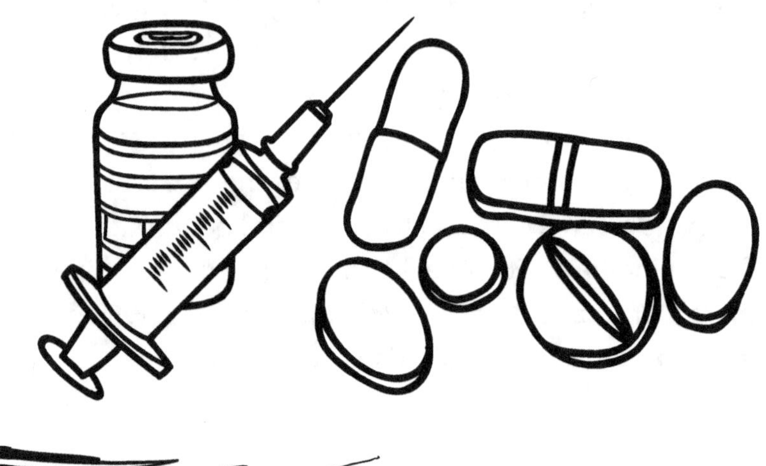

**N. KEHSENI
MARKBRON**

Over the thousands of years that diabetes has been known, scientists and researchers have relentlessly been trying to find a cure for this disease.

Medicines and Treatment

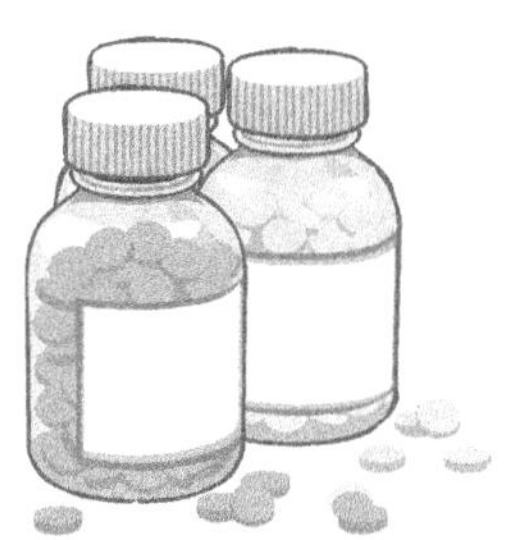

Over the thousands of years that diabetes has been known, scientists and researchers have relentlessly been trying to find a cure for this disease. A lot of remedies were proposed in the 19th and 20th centuries to manage the disease, a lot of which are still used in some parts of the world. In this chapter, we aim to uncover the science behind treatments for diabetes. We equally aim to discuss all the necessary medicines needed to manage the disease and pharmacology (the study of drugs and medicines, including their characteristics, effects, and uses).

For the purpose of education, we will be looking at treatments for both type 1 and type 2 diabetes, but we will focus extensively on the medication and treatment used for type 2 diabetes. Therefore, this chapter will be separated into two parts."

Insulin therapy (insulin infusions)

When we look at type 1 diabetes patients, we see that the underlying cause of their diabetes is due to the fact that the beta cells of their pancreas responsible for producing insulin have been destroyed, and as such, insulin is absent in their system, causing glucose to build up in the blood streams.

In order to remedy this problem, insulin has to be administered to these type 1 diabetes patients. How is insulin produced?

Production of insulin by Recombinant DNA technology

In the early 1920s, scientists Frederick Banting, Charles Best, and

John Macleod discovered insulin's role in regulating blood sugar levels. They extracted insulin from the pancreases of dogs and used it to successfully treat diabetes in humans. After the successful use of insulin in humans, researchers began extracting insulin from the pancreases of animals, particularly pigs and cows, due to their similar insulin structures to human insulin. But this process was labor-intensive, and the yield of insulin from each animal was relatively low.

However, with advancements in biotechnology, insulin can now be produced on large scales using recombinant DNA technology.

Note: Recombinant DNA technology, also known as genetic engineering or gene splicing, involves the manipulation of DNA molecules to create new combinations of genetic material. This technology allows scientists to insert, delete, or modify specific genes within an organism's genome, resulting in the production of desired proteins or the alteration of certain traits.

The basic idea of this recombinant DNA technology in the case of insulin production is to produce a large amount of insulin using a bacteria. We know that bacteria replicate at a very fast rate, and as such, the idea is to get the bacteria to somehow produce insulin while it is replicating.

Here's a simplified breakdown of the process:

- **Isolating the insulin gene:** Scientists identify and isolate the gene that codes for insulin in the cell's DNA. This gene carries the instructions for making insulin.
- **Creating Recombinant DNA:** The isolated insulin gene, through a series of steps, is inserted into a plasmid, which is a small, circular piece of DNA commonly found in bacteria. This creates what's called recombinant DNA, which contains the insulin gene along with other genetic elements necessary for replication and expression.

- **Inserting the recombinant DNA into host cells**: The recombinant DNA is introduced into bacterial cells, such as Escherichia coli (E. coli), which act as tiny factories for producing insulin. This is often done using a process called transformation.
- **Replication and expression**: Once inside the bacterial cells, the recombinant DNA replicates along with the bacterial DNA during cell division. As a result, the bacterial cells start producing insulin based on the instructions encoded by the inserted insulin gene.
- **Harvesting insulin**: The bacterial cells are grown in large fermentation tanks under controlled conditions, providing them with the nutrients they need to multiply and produce insulin. Once a sufficient amount of insulin has been produced, the bacterial cells are harvested, and the insulin is purified from the cell culture.
- **Final purification and formulation**: The harvested insulin undergoes several purification steps to remove impurities and ensure its purity and safety for human use. It is then formulated into various insulin products, such as insulin injections or insulin pens, for use by individuals with diabetes.

Medications Used For Type 1 Diabetes

Insulin and its analogs

Now that we have established that insulin is the main treatment used by type 1 diabetes patients, let's discuss the different types of insulin and how they work.

Now, insulin is a polypeptide. (A polypeptide is a long chain of amino acids (proteins) linked together by peptide bonds.) and as such, it is susceptible to degradation in the gastrointestinal tract. Therefore, for insulin to be most effective, it is mostly administered by subcutaneous injection.

Insulin is divided into 4 categories, and these are based on how quickly they work and for how long they last in the body.
  • Rapid-acting insulin
Under the rapid-acting insulin, we have **Lispro Aspart Glulisine.** They produce peak effects in as little as 30 minutes and have a duration of action of up to 5 hours.
  • Short-acting insulin
Under short-acting insulin, we have **regular.** It produces a peak effect in about 2 hours and 30 minutes, and it has a duration of action of 4-6 hours.
  • Intermediate-acting insulin
Under intermediate-acting insulin, we have **NPH (Neutral Protamine Hagedorn).** NPH has a peak effect of about 8 hours and a duration of action of 10–16 hours.
  • Long-acting insulin
Under long-acting insulin, we have **Insulin Detemir,** which has a peak effect of 6–8 hours and a duration of action of up to 14 hours. Another long-acting insulin is **Glargine,** and this doesn't have a peak effect due to its steady delivery of insulin for up to 24 hours.

Finally, we have **Degluded,** which also has no peak effect due to the steady delivery of insulin and lasts for over 24 hours.
This long-acting insulin is usually taken once a day by type 1 diabetes patients, and it replaces the functioning of the pancreas. In a normal individual, their pancreas usually secretes tiny bits of insulin throughout the day just to make sure that the body sugar levels are in a normal range. This long-acting insulin therefore replaces this basic function of the pancreas in a type 1 diabetes patient. At this point, many of you may wonder what gives some insulin the ability to act faster than others and the ability to last longer than others.

Insulin, as we earlier mentioned, is a polypeptide, and as such, individual insulin molecules always tend to stick to one another, forming long chains of insulin. This chain of insulin is too large to cross from the skin into the blood stream, and as such, it must separate into individual molecules to be able to pass through the subcutaneous tissue (this is the deepest layer of your skin). It's made up mostly of fat cells and connective tissue) into the blood stream. So, what the researchers did was alter the insulin molecules, making some insulin molecules less likely to stick to one another than others.

The insulin that was altered to stick less to one another resulted in faster absorption and rapid action, as is the case with rapid and short-acting insulin. While those that were made to stick faster to one another formed long chains of insulin and resulted in slow absorption and long-lasting action, as is the case with long-acting insulin.

Side Effects of Insulin

- **Hypoglycemia**: This occurs when blood sugar levels dip too low. Symptoms can include shakiness, dizziness, sweating, confusion, and, in severe cases, loss of consciousness.
- **Weight gain**: Some individuals may experience weight gain as a side effect of insulin therapy, particularly if their blood sugar levels were very high before starting treatment. This is also because insulin's role is to open up the cells for glucose to go in for various metabolic processes. As glucose goes into the cell, it causes weight gain.
- **Injection site reactions**: Redness, swelling, or irritation at the injection site are possible side effects, although they usually subside quickly.
- **Allergic reactions**: While rare, some individuals may be allergic to insulin. Symptoms of an allergic reaction can include itching, rash, or difficulty breathing.

- **Lipohypertrophy**: This refers to fatty lumps that can develop under the skin at injection sites with long-term use of insulin.
- **Hypokalemia**: In some cases, insulin therapy can cause low potassium levels in the blood, which can lead to symptoms like weakness, fatigue, muscle cramps, and irregular heart rhythm.

Oral Medications 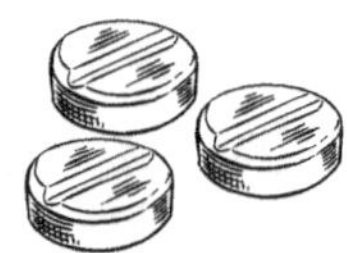

Medications Used for Type 2 Diabetes

In type 2 diabetes, the cells of the body become resistant to the action of insulin, so they take up little or no glucose, and as such, glucose stockpiles in the bloodstream, which can be very detrimental to health, as we have seen throughout. The following are some medications prescribed to type 2 diabetes patients to help lower their blood glucose. It is important to note that all the medicines listed in this book are not medical advice but are for educational purposes only.

Metformin (biguanide):

Metformin is a commonly prescribed medication for treating type 2 diabetes. It acts largely by lowering the quantity of glucose secreted by the liver and improving the sensitivity of muscle cells to insulin. Here's a breakdown of the mechanism and some key medical terms:

1. **Glucose Production Inhibition**: Metformin suppresses gluconeogenesis, which is the process by which the liver produces glucose from non-carbohydrate sources, such as amino acids and glycerol. This action helps lower blood sugar levels by reducing the amount of glucose released into the bloodstream. The term "gluconeogenesis" refers to the generation of new glucose molecules.

2. **Insulin Sensitivity Enhancement**: Metformin improves insulin sensitivity, meaning that it helps cells in the body respond

more effectively to insulin. By enhancing insulin sensitivity, metformin helps glucose enter muscle cells more efficiently, where it can be used for energy production.

Side Effects

The adverse effects of metformin can include gastrointestinal symptoms such as nausea, vomiting, diarrhea, and abdominal discomfort. These side effects are usually mild and transient, but in some cases, they can be bothersome enough to lead to the discontinuation of the medication. Additionally, in rare cases, metformin can cause a serious condition called lactic acidosis, characterized by the buildup of lactic acid in the blood. Lactic acidosis can be life-threatening and requires prompt medical intervention. However, the risk of lactic acidosis with metformin is very low, especially when the medication is used appropriately in individuals without contraindications such as impaired kidney function.

Note

Lactic acidosis is a serious medical condition characterized by an accumulation of lactic acid in the bloodstream. Lactic acid is a byproduct of glucose metabolism (the breakdown of glucose to produce energy) that is normally produced in small amounts and is cleared from the body by the liver. However, in lactic acidosis, either the body produces too much lactic acid or it cannot effectively clear it from the bloodstream.

Symptoms of lactic acidosis can include rapid breathing, confusion, nausea, vomiting, abdominal pain, and an irregular heartbeat. Lactic acidosis is considered a medical emergency and requires prompt treatment to correct the underlying cause and normalize blood pH levels. Left untreated, severe lactic acidosis can lead to organ failure and death.

Sulfonylureas

Sulfonylureas are a class of medications commonly used to treat type 2 diabetes mellitus. Through a series of processes, they stimulate the release of insulin from the beta cells in the pancreas. This mechanism of action helps to lower blood sugar levels by increasing the amount of insulin available to move glucose from the bloodstream into cells for energy production.

There are several types of sulfonylureas used to treat type 2 diabetes, both oral and injectable:

1. Oral sulfonylureas:
    - Glyburide (also known as glibenclamide)
    - Glipizide
    - Gliclazide
    - Tolbutamide
2. Injectable sulfonylureas:
    - Glimepiride

These medications are typically taken once or twice daily, with meals depending on your doctor's prescription, to help control blood sugar levels throughout the day.

Side effects of sulfonylureas may include:

1. Hypoglycemia: One of the most significant risks of sulfonylurea therapy is hypoglycemia, or low blood sugar levels. This can occur if the dose of medication is too high, or if there is inadequate food intake.
2. Weight gain: Some individuals may experience weight gain as a side effect of sulfonylurea treatment.
3. Gastrointestinal disturbances: Sulfonylureas may cause gastrointestinal side effects such as nausea, vomiting, or diarrhea in some individuals.
4. Skin reactions: Rarely, sulfonylureas can cause allergic skin reactions or photosensitivity.

Meglitinides

Meglitinides are another class of medications used to treat type 2 diabetes mellitus. They work by stimulating the release of insulin from the beta cells in the pancreas, similar to sulfonylureas. However, meglitinides have a more rapid onset and shorter duration of action compared to sulfonylureas.

There are two main types of meglitinides commonly prescribed for type 2 diabetes:

1. Repaglinide: Repaglinide is an oral meglitinide medication that is taken before meals to help control blood sugar levels by stimulating insulin release.
2. Nateglinide: Nateglinide is another oral meglitinide medication that is also taken before meals to stimulate insulin secretion from the pancreas.

Side effects of meglitinides may include:

1. Hypoglycemia: Like sulfonylureas, meglitinides can cause hypoglycemia, or low blood sugar levels, particularly if the dose is too high or if meals are skipped.
2. Weight gain: Some individuals may experience weight gain as a side effect of meglitinide therapy.
3. Gastrointestinal disturbances: In some individuals, meglitinides may also cause gastrointestinal side effects such as nausea, vomiting, or diarrhea.
4. Headache: Headache is another possible adverse effect associated with meglitinide use.

As with sulfonylureas, patients taking meglitinides should monitor their blood sugar levels regularly and be educated about the signs and symptoms of hypoglycemia. It's essential to take these medications with meals to reduce the risk of hypoglycemia and to follow healthcare provider instructions regarding dosing.

DPP-4 inhibitors

In order to explain how this drug works, let's take a step back and review a topic we have already discussed. Now, back in the first chapter under type 2 diabetes, we had established that after you eat a meal, a special hormone called GLP-1 (glucagon-like peptide 1) is secreted by the intestines into the bloodstream, and this hormone stimulates the pancreas to produce the right amount of insulin. This GLP-1 equally inhibits the secretion of glucagon, another hormone produced by the pancreas. Glucagon works in opposition to insulin. While insulin lowers blood sugar levels by promoting glucose uptake by cells, glucagon raises blood sugar levels by stimulating the liver to release stored glucose (glycogen) into the bloodstream through a process called glycogenolysis.

Now, there's this special hormone that is secreted by the liver, kidney, intestines, and endothelial cells to inhibit the function of GLP-1, and this hormone is called DPP-4 (dipeptidyl peptidase-4). So, let's say enough insulin has already been secreted into the bloodstream by the action of GLP-1. DPP-4 then comes to tell GLP-1 that enough insulin has already been secreted and it should stop stimulating the pancreas to secrete more insulin. So, it basically inhibits GLP-1's action on the pancreas.

Now, what the researchers did was produce a series of medicines called DPP-4 inhibitors (dipeptidyl peptidase-4 inhibitors). As their name suggests, DPP-4 inhibitors stop the secretion of DPP-4 hormones. If DPP-4 is absent, then GLP-1 will stimulate the pancreas to produce more and more insulin without any obstruction, which will in turn reduce the levels of glucose in the blood.

There are several DPP-4 inhibitors commonly prescribed for type 2 diabetes, all of which are oral medications:

1. Sitagliptin: Sitagliptin is a once-daily DPP-4 inhibitor that helps improve glycemic control by increasing insulin secretion and decreasing glucagon levels.
2. Saxagliptin: Saxagliptin is another once-daily DPP-4 inhibitor that works similarly to sitagliptin in enhancing insulin secretion and reducing glucagon secretion.
3. Linagliptin: Linagliptin is a once-daily DPP-4 inhibitor that has a longer duration of action compared to sitagliptin and saxagliptin, allowing for once-daily dosing without the need for dose adjustments in patients with kidney impairment.

Note

All the medications listed above should be prescribed to you by a health professional. Make sure to take the drugs according to the doctor's prescribed dose.

Side effects of DPP-4 inhibitors may include:

1. Hypoglycemia: While DPP-4 inhibitors generally have a low risk of causing hypoglycemia when used as monotherapy, the risk may increase when combined with other antidiabetic medications that can cause hypoglycemia, such as sulfonylureas or insulin.
2. Nasopharyngitis: According to clinical trials, nasopharyngitis, or inflammation of the nose and throat, is a common side effect of DPP-4 inhibitors.
3. Upper respiratory tract infections: DPP-4 inhibitor use may cause upper respiratory tract infections, including coughs, sore throats, and nasal congestion.
4. Headache is another possible adverse effect of DPP-4 inhibitor therapy.

GLP-1 Agonists

Just like DPP-4 inhibitors, GLP-1 agonists promote the action of

GLP-1 in the secretion of insulin by the pancreas, but they do this differently. A GLP-1 agonist amplifies the action of the GLP-1 hormone, causing an increase in the secretion of insulin by the pancreas. Below are some methods through which GLP-1 agonists work:

1. Stimulating insulin secretion: GLP-1 agonists enhance insulin secretion from the pancreas in a glucose-dependent manner, meaning they increase insulin release when blood sugar levels are high but have little to no effect when blood sugar levels are normal or low.

2. Inhibiting glucagon secretion: GLP-1 agonists suppress the release of glucagon from the pancreas, which helps prevent the liver from producing excess glucose from the conversion of glycogen to glucose, which could further raise blood sugar levels.

3. Slowing gastric emptying: GLP-1 agonists delay the emptying of food from the stomach into the small intestine, which helps regulate the rate at which glucose enters the bloodstream after meals, leading to more stable postprandial (after-meal) blood sugar levels.

4. Increasing satiety: GLP-1 agonists promote feelings of fullness and satiety, which can help reduce food intake and promote weight loss.

There are several GLP-1 agonists available for the treatment of type 2 diabetes, which can be administered either orally or by injection:

Injectable GLP-1 agonists:
- Exenatide: Exenatide is a twice-daily injectable GLP-1 agonist that helps improve glycemic control by mimicking the action of natural GLP-1.
- Liraglutide: Liraglutide is a once-daily injectable GLP-1 agonist that provides sustained blood sugar control and

may also lead to weight loss in some individuals.

- Dulaglutide: Dulaglutide is a once-weekly injectable GLP-1 agonist that offers convenient dosing and can help improve glycemic control and promote weight loss.
- Semaglutide: Semaglutide is available in both once-weekly and once-daily injectable formulations, with the once-weekly formulation demonstrating superior efficacy in lowering blood sugar levels and promoting weight loss.

Oral GLP-1 agonist:

- Semaglutide: In addition to the injectable formulation, semaglutide is also available as an oral tablet taken once daily.

Side effects of GLP-1 Agonists May Include:

1. Gastrointestinal side effects: Common side effects of GLP-1 agonists include nausea, vomiting, diarrhea, and constipation, particularly when starting treatment or increasing the dose. These effects usually improve over time as the body adjusts to the medication.
2. Hypoglycemia: GLP-1 agonists have a low risk of causing hypoglycemia when used as monotherapy. However, the risk may increase when combined with other antidiabetic medications that can cause hypoglycemia, such as sulfonylureas or insulin.
3. Injection site reactions: Injectable GLP-1 agonists may cause injection site reactions, such as redness, swelling, or itching at the injection site.
4. Pancreatitis: Rarely, GLP-1 agonists may increase the risk of pancreatitis, an inflammation of the pancreas. Patients should be monitored for signs and symptoms of pancreatitis, such as severe abdominal pain, nausea, and vomiting, and treatment should be discontinued if pancreatitis is suspected.

SGLT-2 inhibitors (sodium-glucose cotransporter-2 inhibitors)
Somewhere around chapter 3, under the overview of the kidney, we learned that during the filtration process in a normal individual, all the glucose that passes through the kidney is reabsorbed back into the blood stream. However, in a type 2 diabetes patient, not all the glucose is being reabsorbed, as the amount of glucose present is so great that it surpasses the renal threshold (the maximum amount of blood the kidneys can reabsord into the blood streams). The main protein responsible for the reabsorption of glucose from the proximal convoluted tubule (PCT) in the nephron of the kidney into the blood stream is a protein called SGLT-2.

What the researchers did was create a series of medicines called SGLT-2 inhibitors, which, as their names suggest, inhibit the function of SGLT-2, effectively reducing the amount of glucose reabsorbed back into the bloodstream and causing more glucose to pass out as urine. This has the net effect of lowering the amount of glucose in the bloodstream.

There are several SGLT-2 inhibitors Available to Treat Type 2 Diabetes, All of Which are Oral Medications.
1. Canagliflozin: Canagliflozin is an SGLT-2 inhibitor that is taken orally once daily to help lower blood sugar levels by increasing the excretion of glucose in the urine.
2. Dapagliflozin: Dapagliflozin is another oral SGLT-2 inhibitor that is typically taken once daily to reduce blood sugar levels by promoting the elimination of glucose through the urine.
3. Empagliflozin: Empagliflozin is an oral SGLT-2 inhibitor that is usually taken once daily to improve glycemic control by enhancing urinary glucose excretion.
4. Ertugliflozin: Ertugliflozin is a newer oral SGLT-2 inhibitor approved for the treatment of type 2 diabetes. It is also taken

once a day to lower blood sugar levels by increasing urinary glucose excretion.

Side effects of SGLT-2 inhibitors may include:
1. Genital yeast infections: SGLT-2 inhibitors can increase the risk of genital yeast infections, particularly in women. Candida is a type of fungus that naturally exists in the body, usually in balance with other microorganisms. However, in people with diabetes, especially those with uncontrolled blood sugar levels, the elevated glucose levels in bodily fluids, such as urine and vaginal secretions, provide an ideal environment for yeast to multiply. Elevated glucose levels in urine and genital secretions provide an abundant food source for yeast, promoting their growth. Symptoms may include itching, burning, or unusual discharge.
2. Urinary tract infections (UTIs): UTIs are another common side effect of SGLT-2 inhibitor therapy. Symptoms may include painful urination, frequent urination, and lower abdominal pain.
3. Increased urination: Because SGLT-2 inhibitors promote the excretion of glucose in the urine, and because glucose is an osmotic molecule, it attracts water from the surrounding environment to itself through osmosis. SGLT-2 inhibitors can also increase urine output, leading to more frequent urination.
4. Hypotension: Some individuals may experience a decrease in blood pressure upon starting SGLT-2 inhibitor therapy, which can cause symptoms such as dizziness or lightheadedness, particularly when standing up quickly.
5. Dehydration: Increased urine output caused by SGLT-2 inhibitors may lead to dehydration, especially if adequate fluid intake is not maintained.

Alpha-Glucosidase Inhibitors

Whenever you eat a meal rich in glucose, it goes down your digestive tract in a form known as oligosaccharides. This is basically the precursor form of glucose that has not yet been broken down into its monosaccharide derivatives. You can think of oligosaccharides as small groups of friends holding hands. Each friend represents a sugar molecule, and together they form a little chain. Just like how different groups of friends can join hands in different ways, oligosaccharides can have various arrangements of sugar molecules.

An example of an oligosaccharide is lactose, which is found in milk. Lactose is made up of two sugar molecules: glucose and galactose. These two sugar molecules can be arranged in different ways to form lactose. In one arrangement, glucose is linked to galactose in a specific order, while in another arrangement, they can be linked in the opposite order. Both arrangements are still lactose, but they have different structures due to the different ways the sugar molecules are connected. This is essentially what we call an oligosaccharide.

Now, when you eat a meal rich in oligosaccharide glucose, a type of oligosaccharide that contains glucose molecules in a chain, this oligosaccharide needs to be broken down into individual glucose molecules before it is absorbed into the bloodstream. In fact, all oligosaccharides must be broken down before absorption is possible. The breakdown of these oligosaccharides happens in the small intestine by an enzyme called alpha-glucosidase. After this enzyme breaks down the oligosaccharides into their different sugar molecules, like glucose, they are then ready to be absorbed by the small intestine into the bloodstream.

Now, what researchers did was create a list of medications known as alpha-glucosidase inhibitors that inhibit the action of the alpha-glucosidase enzyme, thereby delaying the breakdown, digestion, and absorption of carbohydrates into the blood stream. This leads to a slower and more gradual rise in blood sugar levels after meals, helping to control postprandial (after-meal) glucose spikes.

Common types of alpha-glucosidase inhibitors include acarbose (oral) and miglitol (oral). These medications are typically taken orally, usually before meals.

Adverse effects of acarbose can include gastrointestinal symptoms such as flatulence, diarrhea, abdominal discomfort, and bloating. These effects occur because undigested carbohydrates reach the colon and are fermented by gut bacteria, leading to the production of gas and osmotic effects that cause these symptoms.

Thiazolidinediones (TZDs)

Thiazolidinediones (TZDs) are a class of oral antidiabetic medications used to treat type 2 diabetes mellitus. They work primarily by improving insulin sensitivity in peripheral tissues, such as muscle and fat cells.

The mechanism of action of TZDs involves activation of peroxisome proliferator-activated receptor gamma (PPARγ) in target tissues. PPARγ is a nuclear receptor that plays a key role in regulating genes involved in glucose and lipid metabolism. When activated by TZDs, PPARγ increases the transcription of genes involved in insulin action, resulting in improved insulin sensitivity. This leads to better glucose uptake by peripheral tissues, decreased hepatic glucose production, and overall improvement in glycmic control.

Common types of TZDs include:
- **Rosiglitazone**: An oral medication.
- **Pioglitazone**: Another oral medication.

Adverse effects of thiazolidinediones may include weight gain, fluid retention leading to edema, and an increased risk of heart failure, especially in patients with pre-existing cardiovascular disease. In some studies, pioglitazone has been linked to an increased risk of bladder cancer, although the evidence is not conclusive. Additionally, TZDs can cause liver enzyme elevations, so regular monitoring of liver function is recommended during treatment.

Amylin Analogs

Amylin analogs are a class of medications used to treat type 1 and type 2 diabetes mellitus. They mimic the action of amylin, a hormone produced by the beta cells of the pancreas along with insulin. Amylin helps regulate blood sugar levels by slowing gastric emptying, reducing postprandial glucagon secretion, and promoting satiety.

The main amylin analog used in clinical practice is pramlintide. Pramlintide is a synthetic analog of human amylin and is administered by subcutaneous injection before meals to patients with type 1 or type 2 diabetes who are using insulin therapy.

The main type of amylin analog prescribed in hospitals for type 1 and type 2 diabetes is:
- **Pramlintide:** This is an injectable medication administered subcutaneously before meals to help control postprandial blood sugar levels.

Adverse effects of amylin analogs may include hypoglycemia (especially when used in conjunction with insulin), nausea, vomiting, and injection site reactions. Nausea is a common side effect, particularly when initiating therapy, but it often improves with continued use. To minimize the risk of hypoglycemia, the dose of insulin may need to be reduced when initiating pramlintide therapy.

All the medications listed in this chapter may be used alone or in combination with other diabetes drugs to help manage blood sugar levels. If you suspect you have diabetes, don't just go about taking the medication listed above. It is important to note that every medication listed in this chapter and throughout this book is strictly for educational purposes **ONLY**.

Note:
CONSULT WITH A HEALTHCARE PROFESSIONAL FOR PROPER GUIDANCE AND TREATMENT OPTIONS, AS WELL AS A DETAILED PRESCRIPTION.

Conclusion

"In concluding this journey through 'Diabetes Type 2 Made Simple,' it's not just about what you've learned, but how you've embraced the knowledge within these pages. Throughout our exploration of Type 2 Diabetes, simplicity has been our guiding principle, illuminating the path forward amidst the complexities of managing this condition.

Diabetes management is not a one-size-fits-all approach. It's about finding what works best for you and making informed decisions about your health. By understanding the science behind diabetes and the treatments available, you can take an active role in your healthcare and work collaboratively with your medical team.

Remember, every small step you take towards better management of your diabetes is a victory. Celebrate these successes and learn from any setbacks. Don't underestimate the value of community and support. Connect with others who are on a similar journey, engage with support groups, and lean on your loved ones. Knowledge, coupled with support, can significantly enhance your quality of life.

Thank you for allowing this book to be a part of your journey. My hope is that it has provided you with valuable insights that make living with Type 2 diabetes easier. Your health is a precious asset, and with the right knowledge and support, you can lead a fulfilling and healthy life.
Wishing you strength, resilience, and success on your path to better health."
Warm regards,

N. Kehseni Markbron

I Have A Request

Dear Reader,

As we come to the end of our journey through "Diabetes Type 2 Made Simple," we're eager to hear about your experience with the book and how it has impacted your understanding of Type 2 Diabetes. Your feedback is incredibly valuable to us as we strive to continually improve and empower others on their health journeys.

If you found the book informative, inspiring, or helpful in any way, we would be immensely grateful if you could take a moment to share your thoughts in a testimonial. Your words have the power to inspire others who may be facing similar challenges and guide them toward a path of greater understanding and wellness.

Please feel free to share your honest feedback, whether it's a brief comment on what resonated most with you, how the book has influenced your perspective, or any specific changes you've implemented as a result of reading it. Your review not only helps us to improve, but it also assists fellow individuals in making informed decisions. If you're comfortable, please leave your review on Amazon or any other platform where you prefer to share your thoughts.

Thank you for being a part of this journey, and we look forward to hearing from you.

Warm regards,
N. Kehseni Markbron